Myofascial Release Therapy

Other books by Michael Shea

Biodynamic Craniosacral Therapy, Volume One
Biodynamic Craniosacral Therapy, Volume Two
Biodynamic Craniosacral Therapy, Volume Three
Biodynamic Craniosacral Therapy, Volume Four
Biodynamic Craniosacral Therapy, Volume Five

Myofascial Release Therapy

A Visual Guide to Clinical Applications

Michael J. Shea, PhD
with Holly Pinto, LMT, BCTMB

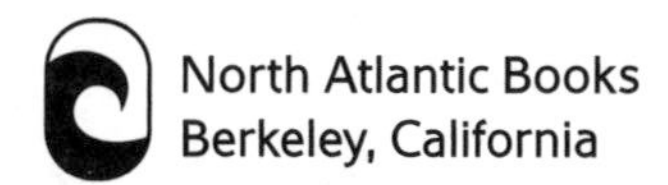
North Atlantic Books
Berkeley, California

Published by
North Atlantic Books
P.O. Box 12327
Berkeley, California 94712

Cover Cover art from *The Three Graces*
by William Edward Frost, 1856
Cover and book design by Jasmine Hromjak
Printed in the United States of America

Myofascial Release Therapy: A Visual Guide to Clinical Applications is sponsored by the Society for the Study of Native Arts and Sciences, a nonprofit educational corporation whose goals are to develop an educational and cross-cultural perspective linking various scientific, social, and artistic fields; to nurture a holistic view of arts, sciences, humanities, and healing; and to publish and distribute literature on the relationship of mind, body, and nature.

North Atlantic Books' publications are available through most bookstores. For further information, visit our website at www.northatlanticbooks.com or call 800-733-3000.

MEDICAL DISCLAIMER: The following information is intended for general information purposes only. Individuals should always see their health care provider before administering any suggestions made in this book. Any application of the material set forth in the following pages is at the reader's discretion and is his or her sole responsibility.

Library of Congress Cataloging-in-Publication Data
Shea, Michael J., 1948- author.
Myofascial release therapy : a visual guide to clinical applications / Michael J. Shea with Holly Pinto.
p. ; cm.
Includes bibliographical references and index.
ISBN 978-1-58394-845-3 (paperback : alk. paper) -- ISBN 978-1-58394-846-0 (ebook)
I. Pinto, Holly, author. II. Title.
[DNLM: 1. Myofascial Pain Syndromes--therapy. 2. Massage--methods. WE 550]
RC925.5
616.7'4206--dc23

2014016920

1 2 3 4 5 6 7 8 UNITED 19 18 17 16 15 14

Printed on recycled paper

Contents

Introduction

Holly Pinto

This manual serves many purposes for today's contemporary therapist. You can use each release found in the manual individually, or you can combine releases based on your assessment of the client and what might be indicated for your session. There are many great models of bodywork out there. Use this manual as another tool to add to your toolbox. It is more important to explore your own belief systems and biases. Then you can transition from one system of work to another staying in the rhythm of the client's nervous system, which in today's chaotic world is extremely important. Creating a safe therapeutic container to provide a skillful therapy session is the goal for a successful session. We hope you find this manual useful.

Michael Shea

I learned a lot about fascia and its manipulation at the Rolf Institute between 1979 and 1982. The work presented in this book, however, is not Rolfing. I highly recommend anyone interested in furthering their knowledge of working with the fascia to take the training at the Rolf Institute in Boulder, Colorado. My clinical practice from the beginning included many orthopedic conditions and children with spastic cerebral palsy. I was not able to apply many of the principles of organization that I learned at the Rolf Institute, and consequently began modifying what I had learned in order to adapt to the needs of my clients, especially all the infants and children I was seeing. At the same time, I was influenced by other systems of fascial manipulation such as from the osteopathic community as well as numerous colleagues working in this field. The term myofascial release comes from the original fascial manipulation developed by the osteopathic community in the early 1950s. This text is about the adaptation I made, and that my dear friend and colleague Holly Pinto has made. It is still valid now as it was when I first practiced and taught it in the 1980s.

The first place I ever taught myofascial release was in the great state of Texas in 1987. Holly Pinto was one of my first students and has continued working with the material I presented, along with integrating her own brilliant clinical skills and knowledge base in myofascial release. I am greatly honored that Holly teaches this work and spent the time to thoroughly adapt this text to the needs of the contemporary client in 2014.

This book is divided into three sections. The first section has to do with anatomy and clinical considerations. The second section comprises a photographic atlas that is thoroughly annotated, so the contemporary therapist can use it immediately in their work. Sections titled "The Work" provide a condensed, quick review of most of the techniques, but are not a substitute for learning this work. It is important that each release is read in full detail. The third and last section is a series of commentaries and essays that I wrote about my clinical experience. While there is some overlap and redundancy within these essays, they were originally intended as a stand-alone information guide to round out a person's knowledge base.

SECTION 1

Theory and Application

CHAPTER 1

Myofascial Release: A Holistic Approach

> *Although myofascial release concepts have been used for many decades, little has been documented or written about them. The system is a complex form of soft tissue manipulation based on the operator's ability to monitor functional, anatomic, and neurologic influences. Developed by American osteopathic therapists, myofascial release led, with important exceptions, to clinically pertinent, fascially-based discussions almost exclusively in the osteopathic literature, but only after 1950.*
> (Ward, 1993, p. 225)

Still today, "the study of fascia and its function as an organ of support has been largely neglected and overlooked for several decades" (Findley & Schleip, 2007, p. 2). Recently, more attention is being placed on fascia and fascial research. The finest researchers and experts in the field of fascia gathered in October 2007 at the first International Fascia Research Congress. It was a sold-out conference in Boston at Harvard Medical School. The second conference was held in Amsterdam in 2009, the third was in Vancouver, British Columbia, in 2012, and a fourth is planned to be held in Washington, DC in September 2015. The focus of these conferences is to present findings on the latest research of the human fasciae system. "The Fascial Research Congress is the first international conference dedicated to fascia in all its forms and functions" (Findley & Schleip, 2007, p. 2).

Myofascial release is usually taught as a positioning technique or stroke intent. As a technique or intention, its primary focus is the soft tissues of the body, especially the fascia. The approaches are either direct techniques, such as Rolfing developed by Dr. Ida Rolf, or indirect techniques, such as muscle energy and strain/counter-strain (Greenman, 1989). When joint biomechanical rules, called arthrokinematics, are integrated into the treatment, the treatment is a myofascial manipulation. The presenting symptoms of the client, the physician's orders, and the evaluation skills of the therapists are combined to determine the techniques used. The continuity of treatment methods and strategies depends upon feedback from the client, clinical observations about the client's physical and emotional demeanor, and the subjective experience of the therapist. Although presenting symptoms and physician's orders are key factors, the background and training of the therapist influences the decision to use direct or indirect techniques.

Regardless of the direct or indirect myofascial techniques chosen, the basic question remains: How should these different techniques be organized for clinical effectiveness? This chapter looks at clinical effectiveness from a holistic point of view. Initially, it will consider the skills, rather than the techniques, of myofascial release. Next, the holistic principles of the fascia connective tissue are presented followed by a review of specific treatment strategies. The final review includes conclusions based on a holistic model. Because a holistic approach to myofascial release is about skills, this chapter starts with skills and ends with skills.

Holistic Skills

Listening to both the verbal and nonverbal aspects of the client's story is a primary skill in a holistic practice of myofascial release. Failure to listen carefully and sensitively leads a therapist to make judgments that are academic and lack subjective understanding of the unique story each client brings to the treatment room. A client's body can inform the therapist about many things that can only be found out by listening to the client's words (Maitland, 1986). Listening at this depth requires a therapist to commit time to the process and to offer belief to even the most subtle remarks. Every word and body movement has purpose as clients unfold their story for the willing therapist.

Listening at this depth requires a therapist to suspend judgment until the story is told. Leaping prematurely to the end with a quick fix negates the client's uniqueness. What is very real for the client may be completely irrelevant for the therapist unless the therapist shifts perception. This skill also includes uncovering meanings held within the client/therapist relationship. Both the therapist and the client have expectations for the therapy, some of which may be unspoken or even unknown at the time. A good question to ask is: What intention does the therapist hold for the relationship and does it match the intention of the client?

Many people feel that communication between people with the same language is fairly automatic and uncomplicated. However, as is well-known, many misunderstandings can occur. Communication is downright frustrating at times between people with different points of view, especially when conversations change and involve numerous concepts and ideas that may be foreign to others. If therapists are to understand the physical problems of their clients, they need to have a quality and depth of appreciation for the complexities surrounding both verbal and nonverbal communication. Paying attention to verbal communication and the links that it has to body sensation and posture is a refined skill in the holistic practice of myofascial release.

The human body has not only an exquisite capacity to adapt and compensate for stress and trauma, but also an inherent capacity to inform. The client's body can provide clues related to the problem that may never be found by the most thorough objective examination. The most common example of this is how often the presenting problem is linked to accidents much earlier in the client's life and/or is coupled to current social and psychological relationships. If someone is being treated for injuries resulting from a motor vehicle accident, a surprising amount of information may be obtained by asking the client where he or she was going to or coming from at the time of the accident. The subtlety and interconnectedness of some of the messages coming from the client can be priceless. From a holistic point of view, the more clients are tuned into their body, the more they will become aware of such subtleties and relatedness. Thus, part of the role of the therapist is to educate the client to notice the little things and to report them to the therapist.

Another key in holistic myofascial release is developing appropriate and insightful skills of observation. Bear in mind that vision is formed by 80 percent of neuroassociation and networking within the brain and only 20 percent from the retinas (Varela, Thompson, & Rosch, 1992). The implications of this may be clinically significant. It is quite possible to have many thoughts triggered by observing clients. Therapists may have theoretical notions about the way a body should look, move, and perform that fail to match the individual client. These preconceptions have the potential to influence the quality of the clinical work both consciously and unconsciously. Thus, skills of observation include looking at the client holistically. That is, seeing him or her as a whole person rather than a group of symptoms and being clear that the thoughts and ideas triggered by observing the client belong to the therapist, rather than the client.

Observation skills may alter the way myofascial release is practiced. Holistic observation skills are based on the self reflection of the therapist, with careful attention being paid to the therapist's sensations, feelings, and inner thoughts as he or she begins to resonate with the client. Heisenberg stated in his uncertainty principle that one cannot observe something without changing it. Is it possible that looking at a client in a clinical mode could change him or her? Meaning is uncovered by paying attention to the moment-to-moment experience occurring not only within the client's body and state of mind, but also in the body and mind of the therapist. Therapeutic clarity arises from this quality of attention, which is often referred to as presence and grounding.

Therapists have many nonclinical thoughts about the client (this person is attractive, this person looks sad, etc.) and about themselves (I'm tired, I'd like to go home, etc.). These nonclinical thoughts and associated sensations are usually considered an epiphenomenon (Sheets-Johnstone, 1992). Sensations and feelings are subjective and are often discarded as having little relevance to the client-therapist relationship in a treatment session. However, personal thoughts and feelings are important and have an impact upon the relationships therapists have with their clients. This involves the psychological issues of transference and countertransference between the therapist and the client. The self-reflection of the therapist helps determine the quality, quantity, depth, and duration of touch. For example, therapists may be distracted by events in their personal lives. Sometimes these distractions are carried into the treatment room and may cause a loss of attention on the part of the therapist and thus affect the quality of touch and the treatment outcome.

Related to the skills of observation is the development of a therapeutic sense of how clients hold their unique bodily experience. This sense is based in the aesthetics of balance, form, and shape. Of particular importance are observations of symmetry and of the pattern of nervous system arousal, settling, and resolution. Understanding the three-dimensional aesthetics of balance, form, and shape requires the development of seeing with soft eyes or wide angle viewing.

One mode of learning how to treat a client is through observing the symmetry or lack of symmetry in their musculoskeletal system. Symmetry is first and foremost a result of embryological development around a midline. The therapist looks at a client and notices that one shoulder is higher, one leg is shorter, one hip is higher, or the head is not on the midline. From an embryological and developmental point of view, the body was not designed to be symmetrical (Blechschmidt & Gasser, 1978). All bodies have intrinsic, natural, right-left, front-back, top-bottom splits in their symmetry (Dychtwald, 1977). The body actually develops in a spiral pattern that mimics the double helix pattern of DNA and RNA (Dart, 1950) around a midline. Rather than look at symmetry, the holistic therapist looks at the total form and balance of the client's body. This requires a different kind of vision.

Observing the lack of symmetry may or may not provide accurate information about clients' orthopedic trauma. However, looking more closely at the background of the client's body helps develop what is called soft seeing. Soft seeing is a skill the therapist uses to track the client's central, autonomic, and enteric nervous systems and the role that these systems have in mediating stress and shock/trauma in the client's fascia. Soft seeing includes observing skin color, postural tone, rapid eye movements, patterns of muscular contraction, micromovements (fasciculations) such as shaking and trembling, changes in breathing, voice patterns, sweating, and so on. These signals indicate arousal of the sympathetic nervous system. The client may be experiencing an affect or imprinting coming from their held states of stress and trauma (Levine, 1997).

The sympathetic and parasympathetic are the two major divisions of the autonomic nervous system. Clinically, sympathetic nervous system arousal is supposed to be coupled into the parasympathetic nervous system (Siegel, 1999). This means that both systems are designed to function reciprocally. The parasympathetic nervous system raises its tone as the client's vagal brake attempts to lower sympathetic nervous system arousal (Porges, Doussard-Roosevelt, & Maiti, 1994). The therapist observes the client's individual style of autonomic nervous system cycling from activation and arousal to settling and resolution. This observation of autonomic nervous system cycling will produce more clinically efficient outcomes from myofascial release. The therapist will be able to pace the input of the manipulation to match the autonomic nervous system style of the client. Soft seeing starts the moment a client walks in for the appointment and lasts throughout the treatment as the therapist concurrently tracks autonomic nervous system activity.

Recognition of sympathetic nervous system arousal is clinically important, as overexcitement of the sympathetic nervous system leads to hyperarousal and greatly diminishes the effectiveness of myofascial release. Clinical signs of sympathetic nervous system activation can readily be seen regardless of whether the client is sitting, standing, or lying on the treatment table. These autonomic patterns are effects from stress and shock/trauma. They can be integrated by acknowledging them verbally and kinesthetically by slowing the technique and lightening the touch. Small spontaneous client fasciculations are verbally acknowledged by the therapist. What is important in these micromovements is for the client to become aware of the movement and to allow the arising sensation to occur without judgment or interference. This permits integration to occur between the myofascial and the autonomic nervous systems and avoids retraumatizing the client (Levine, 1997).

One goal of holistic myofascial release is to encourage clinicians to see their clients with new eyes and new hands. The clinician can view each client as a whole person, rather than just their exterior asymmetries and complaints. The therapist appreciates the client's unspoken message regarding his or her inner emotional and social circumstances. Recognizing that the client from a different cultural background may be embarrassed at being seen in his or her underwear, for example, impacts the treatment. This embarrassment or confusion may be an opportunity for the clinician to change approaches and help the client to relax, and for the therapist to do what is appropriate and correct for that client. Safety and trust are essential ingredients to a successful therapeutic outcome.

Holistic myofascial release looks at the ways the client has structured his or her past experience as it shows itself in the body.

Myofascial release offers the possibility to destructure past somatic experience and to reform or create a new structure. When the client's contact with the world is thwarted by orthopedic injury, shock/trauma, stress, and so on, the inner world of the body becomes distorted. A central focus of holistic practice is to rearrange these distorted myofascial patterns. One of the goals of this approach is to help clients experience the interconnectedness between the experience of their bodies from the inside and its relationship to the outside world. This includes how sensations, feelings, and emotions are organized in the body and how they are coupled to meaning and memory (Pert, 1997). To know how the fascia shapes itself from inner and outer experience is important to the understanding of myofascial release (Keleman, 1986).

To review, these are some of the elements of practicing myofascial release holistically: the first is to acknowledge personal thoughts and feelings and then to become centered and grounded by paying attention to the present moment. The second element is appreciating the uniqueness of the whole client by carefully listening and observing. The third element relates to the aesthetics of balance, form, and shape of how the client holds experience in his or her body, especially with the autonomic nervous system. Myofascial release is an art form, and the therapist is a sculptor. These foundational skills form the basis for organizing a treatment plan for the client. This is the beginning of a holistic understanding of myofascial release.

Holistic Aspects of Fascia

When practicing myofascial release holistically, it is important to understand some biological principles and systemic characteristics of the fascial system. The first principle is that fascia is an organic crystal with an electrical, chemical, and magnetic communication system (Oschman, 1993a). An orthopedic injury, stress, or shock/trauma to the body changes this bioelectromagnetic configuration at the cellular level. Compression of a crystalline substance, such as fascia, produces a change in the electrical field of the tissue. Change produced by compression of the crystalline lattice of the fascia is called the piezoelectric effect. Fascia is a semiconductor. Thus myofascial release may change or enhance this bioelectromagnetic configuration because direct compression of the fascia is often employed in myofascial release. Even though there is much research to be done in this field, it is known that enhancing the bioelectromagnetic configuration will increase circulation, which speeds up tissue healing response time (Rubik et al., 1994).

Second, there is a continuous fascial sheath surrounding every muscle, organ, and bone of the body. In addition, the superficial fascia is one continuous layer of fascia that is subdermal. The retinaculum of the feet and ankle contain thick fascial bands that form a bridge between the deep and superficial fasciae of the body. The fibers in connective tissue fascia include collagen, elastin, and reticulum (Oschman, 1984). There are four categories of collagen fibers. Type I is found in loose, dense connective tissue, which is the most commonly treated type of fascia. Type II collagen is found in hyaline cartilage. Type III collagen is found in the fetal dermis and lining of the arteries. Type IV collagen is found in the basement membrane of cells (Grodin & Cantu, 1992). A continuum of structure and communication travels from every cell nucleus in the body via the microtubules within the cell through the basement membrane wall to the collagen fibers of the fascia itself (Grodin & Cantu, 1992). This implies that myofascial release may affect the client's body systemically, not just locally. The therapist needs to be able to observe the whole body of the client and the interrelationship of the fascia to the autonomic nervous system, which directly innervates the fascia.

The third biological principle related to all connective tissue is concerning the ground substance. Ground substance is a viscous, amorphous solution with high water content. Ground substance contains collagen fibers and other cells, especially the fibroblasts.

Histologically, the fibroblasts are the primary secretory cells in connective tissue, existing in the collagen, elastin, and reticular fibers, as well as the ground substance. It is a function of the ground substance to diffuse nutrients and process waste products. The ground substance also acts as a mechanical barrier to invading bacteria and other microorganisms. Together the various collagen fibers and ground substance are called the extracellular matrix (Grodin & Cantu, 1992).

The primary components of ground substance are glycosaminoglycans substances and water. Glycosaminoglycans substances were formally referred to as acid mucopolysaccharides. They can be divided into sulfated and nonsulfated groups. The nonsulfated group, which is predominantly hyaluronic acid, binds water. Connective tissue is approximately 70 percent water. A change in the water content of the connective tissue affects the critical interfiber distance in the ground substance. When there is an injury to the soft tissue, the ground substance appears dehydrated, and the collagen fibers bind together to form a gel-sol relationship. In an orthopedic trauma or in related stress to the fascial system, the dehydration of the ground substance causes the interfiber distance between the collagen fibers to shorten. This dehydration causes the ground substance to become like a glue or gel. The collagen fibers begin to crosslink and form a much tighter bond to protect the body. Myofascial release and purposeful movement have the potential to rehydrate the ground substance, which causes it to revert back into solution. This subsequently returns the collagen to a healthy interfiber distance. This is what is meant by the gel-sol relationship. Clinically, around the area of injury, the skin and fascia feel tight and dry. Then with appropriate manipulation, the tissue returns to buoyancy and flexibility. All of these changes in the ground substance are mediated by the bioelectromagnetic configuration of the fascia.

The fourth principle is that fascia acts like a fluid system in response to stress and strain. Stress and strains on living biological material are described by the field of biorheology in terms such as shear forces and tension. Fascia exhibits non-Newtonian-type fluid/semi-solid, chaotic behavior because of the tensile properties of collagen. Stress to the fascial system may be unpredictable in its effects. Injury to the fascial system causes systemic compensations throughout the body, not just locally. It is difficult to predict where compensatory patterns will occur (Feitis & Schultz, 1996). Somato-visceral and viscero-somatic interactions are not in register segmentally in the spinal cord (Patterson & Howell, 1989). Visceral input converges on the cord along with somatic afferents may influence the entire spinal cord and brain as one homogenous neuronal pool rather than limiting itself to discrete segments of the spinal cord (Willard & Patterson, 1992). This leaves many possibilities for systemic effects from something as simple as joint pain in the knee. Multiple referral sites from acute and chronic nerve root irritation are distributed through the body, not just in the fascial system. Chronic knee pain may adversely affect the bladder, liver problems can affect the eyes, and so on.

Nociception, the processing of pain, has a pervasive influence in the body and central nervous system. Nociceptive mechanisms both locally and centrally contribute to the adaptive response. Thus a minor injury to a part of the body that is already under stress may push the whole system over the edge causing a reaction quite larger than normal (Willard & Patterson, 1992). For example, a client may have a subclinical bowel problem such as intermittent constipation, then sprain their ankle and develop headaches, lose sleep, and enter a period of chronic pain from seemingly innocuous events.

The fifth principle is that the body is capable of building more fascia than it can remove. Scientists feel that the need for rapid, adaptive patterning is part of the evolutionary process (Oschman, 1993a). Any injury to the soft tissues of the body undergoes a process of shortening and tightening to heal. These changes in collagenous binding begin to occur within 20 minutes of an injury or sustained postural distortion. The longer the distorted, immobile position is maintained, the more the collagen fibers will crosslink to form newer, tighter bonds. These bonds will continue to proliferate over time to adjacent joints above and below the site of the injury. Fascial binding affects the entire body because the fascia has multilayered continuity from top to bottom and outside to in. This accounts for some of the reflex activity seen in myofascial pain syndromes (Travell & Simons, 1992). Recognition of how the whole body fascial system compensates or adapts to trauma and injuries is an important treatment consideration with myofascial release.

Treatment Strategies

At a practical level for time management during a myofascial release treatment, the superficial fascia is engaged for the first 20 to 30 minutes, followed by the deep fascia for 10 to 15 minutes. This is followed at the end of the treatment by coming back out to the superficial fascia layer and organizing the part of it known as the integrative fascia, which surrounds the erector spinae muscles. The integrative fascia is all the paraspinal fascia. Organizing the paraspinal fascia has a direct and positive biomechanical effect on the brain and spinal cord via the denticulate ligaments and its dural connections. This includes the vascular and lymphatic vessels of the spine known as Batson's plexus. These central midline elements relay tissue changes, occurring throughout the body, both biomechanically and neurologically directly into the spinal cord and brain.

When multiple treatment sessions are possible for a single client, three session units may be organized. Several options are available when viewing a series of three treatments as a unit of work. One triad might begin with a session on the lower extremities and pelvic girdle, followed by a second session on the shoulder girdle and upper extremities, then a third session specific to the axial midline and spine. Other triads might focus on three sets of three sessions: three superficial fascia sessions, followed by three deep fascia release sessions, concluding with three paraspinal integrative sessions. The combinations possible with this triad model are numerous.

There are three additional practical organizational concepts. The first is that the dorsal and ventral fasciae of the trunk migrate laterally under stress or from injury. This is a clinical observation from numerous therapists. This means that in the myofascial release treatment, the therapist moves the fascia over the abdomen and rib cage up and back toward the spinal column to restore postural tone. Then the fascia over the spinal erectors is moved medially and down from trapezius to sacrum. Quite simply the therapist lifts the ventral fasciae up the front and drops the ventral fasciae down the back.

Strategies for manipulating fascial restrictions are based on the functional divisions of the fascial system and how appropriate contact is made with this system. These divisions are called the deep and superficial fascia. The easiest way to engage the system is at the level of the superficial fascia and the coverings of the superficial postural support muscles. After freedom is achieved in the superficial layers and enlivened with broad light contact, the deep fascia is engaged (Rolf, 1989). The deep fascia is the layer continuous with and surrounding the deep postural support muscles. These muscles include the tibialis and peroneal group in the lower extremity, the interosseous membrane between the tibia and the fibula, the adductor complex, the ilio-psoas-diaphragm group, the mediastinum, the pectoralis minor and subscapularis, the scalenes, the pterygoid muscles, and the meninges.

Second, the myofascial release therapist accesses the superficial fascia of the client along the coronal plane of the body while the client is side lying. The coronal plane is like a tailor's seam on the lateral side of a suit or pair of pants. It is the point where many fascial planes converge, such as the aponeurosis of the abdominal fascia and the lumbar fascia. The osseous margins like the iliac crest are ideal places to differentiate fascial layers as they converge at the coronal plane. Key structures to free with myofascial release are the lateral malleolus, head of the fibula, greater trochanter, crest of the ileum, the ribs, the head of the humerus, the mastoid process of the temporal bones, the parietal (bone) ridges, and the occipital squama.

Third, the therapist works with the intention to separate the fascial septa between the muscles that are not gliding over each other properly. The fascial septa are the bags or containers of the individual muscles. Injury causes the septa to bind or glue to each other via the gel-sol relationship of the ground substance, thus restricting motion. In addition, myofascial release includes work on the various retinacula on the legs, arms, trunk, and spine. It is the belief of this author that the posterior serratus muscles act as retinacula for the erectors. The retinaculi have significant potential for binding because the superficial and deep fasciae merge at each of the retinaculum. Releasing these deep and superficial fascial junctions is essential for free movement of the fascia and postural alignment.

An important treatment component of myofascial release is disengagement. As the therapist applies direct pressure to the client's body, it is important for the therapist to periodically (approximately every 3 minutes) take their hands off the client's body and observe their respiration for a minimum of two or three cycles. This allows the client to integrate the treatment into their autonomic nervous system and permits the therapist to evaluate the cumulative effect of their treatment. Without periodic disengagement or proper pacing of the work, the risk of retraumatizing the client increases as the autonomic nervous system fails to cycle properly (Levine, 1997). The central and autonomic nervous systems take longer to integrate changes in the soft tissue from myofascial release.

During disengagement, it is an ideal time to visually scan the client from head to toe. Close attention is paid to the eyes, skin color, postural tone, facial expression, set of the jaw, tension patterns in the scalenes, capital flexion of the head, position of the trunk (elevated or depressed), shaking or trembling in the extremities, contraction in the rectus abdominis, and so forth. These are indications of sympathetic nervous system arousal. Usually these signals are a message for the therapist to slow down and take a longer break between the applications of contact and pressure. This is an excellent time to request feedback from the client regarding the quality of touch or by simply asking if the client is comfortable. Therapists may also pay attention to how clients respond with affect such as involuntary body movement and the tone of it. Asking a client where they are sensing the work rather than how they are feeling the work is an important distinction. Feeling may be a loaded word for clients. Helping the client to reassociate to body sensation is a valuable rule of thumb in myofascial release. In addition, use of the word allow gives the client freedom to explore their experience, that is, "Can you allow this sensation to move into your back?," "Can you allow this sensation to move into your hip?," and so forth.

Chronically immobile, frozen tissue may be indicative of shock and/or trauma (Levine, 1997). Tissue that has a waxy flexibility (finger pressure that leaves a white indentation in the tissue for several minutes), or tissue that has low tone may also be an indication of shock and/or trauma. During shock and/or trauma, the organism has two other choices when flight or fight is thwarted. One choice is called inhibitory freezing. The body becomes rigid and stiff with fear. This freezing response in governed by the amygdala, which is the deepest part of the limbic system or emotional brain. Soft tissue shortens and decreases circulation (Levine, 1992). When left untreated, this condition armors the body by stiffening in discreet patterns (Reich, 1945).

Another choice the body makes from shock and/or trauma is called resignation. This response is hardwired into the nervous system and is seen quite often in the animal world. It is known as playing possum. The body collapses into a defenseless posture, and the soft tissue becomes hypotonic. This condition also has psychological correlates and usually is seen in endogenous depression

(Herman, 1997). Together these two conditions frequently habituate into the myofascial system. The myofascial system responds best to manipulation that is slow, quiet, thoughtful, and well-paced. Holistic myofascial release palpation skills are based on quality, quantity, depth, direction, and duration as mentioned earlier. As Ida Rolf once said, "Take the tissue into its anatomically correct position and ask for movement." This movement facilitates a deeper integration of the nervous system as the fascia reorganizes. It also reduces the occasional perception of pain when the manipulation touches a sensitive area of the client's body. Asking the client to breathe into the point of contact is always appropriate. Slow, purposeful movement participation by the client is critical in restoring the function of hypotonic tissues. Clinical failures often result from a lack of engaging the client consciously. A morphic focus used with hypertonicity seems relatively ineffective compared with a tonal focus for hypotonic tissue.

Review and Conclusion

The hallmark of myofascial release is a sequence of intentions and bodily awareness that includes contact with the client's breath and soliciting active movement. This includes focused attention by the therapist with his or her own body and mind, verbal interaction, and finally integration and closure of the treatment. Contact with the client begins preverbally and intuitively as he or she makes the appointment, which generates thoughts and feelings in the therapist. Contact includes carefully listening and observing a client's history. The flow of the contact moves to a stage of palpating the tissue itself when the client is in the treatment room.

Next, the therapist observes the client's breathing. Asking the client to breathe slowly and deeply into the point of contact allows integration in the autonomic nervous system and permits the client to feel in control of the session. Different breathing patterns indicate arousal of the sympathetic nervous system. Therapists may sense their own breath and be aware of any changes in their own respiratory pattern as a way of staying grounded and present for the client. This creates resonance between the neurological systems of the client and therapist (Siegel, 1999). The therapist's respiration is an important feedback system about not only their own internal states, but also those of the client through a type of perceptual transference.

Throughout these stages of contact, the client has the opportunity to develop awareness of their individual pattern of tension and holding. As this somatic awareness is enhanced, the possibility for stress reduction and a reassociation to body comfort and ease is possible. It is something generated from the inside of the client with the skill of the therapist acting as a guide. Reassociation to sensation ultimately uncouples the shock and trauma from the client's injury and creates an organized, meaningful experience (Perls, 1951). It is essential to cultivate bodily awareness and uncoupled shock and trauma from tissue effects by attending to sensations. The therapist models this attention for the client, and thus mirrors a much deeper level of integration and functionality for the client. This may simply mean that clients walk better at the end of the treatment or that they have just released a month's worth of tension, simply because they had an insight during the treatment about how they hold their tension.

It is difficult to predict where the client will work with their subjective body awareness. This is when the therapist's skill with myofascial release comes into play. Intervention is being made with a complex pattern that the client has formed in his or her fascia and nervous systems. This pattern has a significant relationship to other systems of the body, as well as the sociocultural context within which the client currently lives. Intervention in the fascial system has the potential to impact many levels of a client's life. Understanding basic principles and skills, plus allowing subjective somatic insights rather than merely applying a technique, offers an opportunity for more successful clinical outcomes.

This is a holistic model of myofascial release. The evolution of experienced meaning for clients is impacted by their body, their sense of self, the social context in which they live, and, at a very pragmatic level, by the therapist's pacing, depth, and direction of touch. These qualities of a holistic model help reduce the impersonal, distant, and cold affect of therapists and physicians that clients so often complain about. The client is empowered when the therapist models empathic contact and is sensitive to the whole client. The therapist is able to resonate with the client and vice versa. Myofascial release becomes a collaborative event.

Holistic myofascial release requires personal awareness and subtle observation skills on the part of the therapist. The client needs to be verbally empowered to tell the therapist when to stop, when to slow down, and when to back off. This is called the rule of stop. Therefore, it is important to carefully educate the client about reassociation to their subjective sensations, images, and thoughts rather than ignoring or suppressing them. Of primary importance in the holistic model is therapeutic insight, emotional clarity, and sensitivity on the part of the therapist (Johnson, 1986).

Proper contact is the key to myofascial release. Contact is more than just talking with and touching the client. Making unbiased, unconditional, nonjudgmental contact with the whole client is essential in holistic practice. These treatment principles are the foundation for how to see and touch the client. Myofascial release is the medium. The message is located in the therapist's own thoughts, feelings, images, and sensations; the coldness or warmth evoked by the client; and the understanding of such responses in dealing with the client (Keleman, 1986). The end result clinically is a more rapid healing response to injured tissue and the possibility for meaning to arise in the client.

> *To be in contact, we need to be grounded, have adequate boundaries, enjoy unrestricted breathing, have access to feeling, and have the intention to be present. To be fully present, reflects a functional and durable sense of self.*
> (Conger, 1994, p. 56)

This article originally appeared in The Clinical Bulletin of Myofascial Therapy, Vol. 2, No. 1, published by the Haworth Medical Press. It was called "Myofascial Release: Blending the Orthopedic and Somatic Models." It was coauthored by Dale Keyworth, PT.

CHAPTER 2

Fascial Anatomy and Microphysiology Simplified

Histological Makeup and Classification of Connective Tissue

Types of Connective Tissue

Dense regular
Dense irregular
Loose irregular

Components

Cells (fibroblasts): Synthesize collagen and ground substance (Cousins are chondroblast and osteoblast)
Extracellular matrix

Extracellular Matrix (FIBERS)

Collagen

- Type I: Ordinary tissue (loose tissue) and bone
- Type II: Hyaline cartilage
- Type III: Fetal dermis, arteries
- Type IV: Basement membranes

Elastin:

Lines the arteries

Reticulin:

Supports glands and lymph nodes

Extracellular Matrix (Ground Substance)

Ground substance

Viscous gel with much water content

Substance in which collagen lies

Purpose

Diffusion of nutrients and waste products

Determines to some extent the histological characteristics of the tissue

Maintains critical interfiber distance

More abundant in early life—decreased with age

Mechanical barrier against bacteria

Components

- Glycosaminoglycan's lubricating effect, maintain cruticalinterfiber distance, minimize collagen crosslinking
- Proteoglycans; primarily bind water

Types of Connective Tissue

Dense regular

- Aponeurosis
- Joint capsules
- Periosteum

- Dermis of skin
- Fascial sheaths (in areas of mechanical stress)

Loose irregular

- Superficial fascial sheaths
- Nerve sheaths (support sheaths of internal organs)
- Muscle
- Thin meshwork of collagen

The fasciae of the body appear as wrappings that cover the viscera, the muscles, and the bones. The fascial wrapping around the bones is called periosteum. The fascial bags in which the various organs and viscera are enveloped are called subserous fascia. The subcutaneous fascial bag that invests the entire body, from head to foot, is called superficial fascia—one continuous layer of fascia. Every muscle is invested in a fascial bag, beginning in the embryo. The organs develop in the fascial bags. Therefore, the body develops and is defined by the fascial bags and the fascial tubes of the alimentary, dural, and cardiovascular systems (Oschman, 1989a, 1989b; Oschman, 1990).

There is a whole system of interconnecting tubes that are made of connective tissue fascia—the whole arterial system. The alimentary system is a sequence of three different fascial tubes that start at the mouth and end at the anus. The meninges invest the brain and connect to the paraspinal fasciae via the denticulate ligaments. There is an interrelating system of fascial planes that connect one muscle group to another. For instance, over the leg is the crural fascia that merges at the inguinal ligament with the transversalis fascia that envelopes the whole peritoneal cavity. The transversalis fascia comes up and merges with the diaphragmatic fascia, which merges with the parietal pleura around the lungs, and the parietal pleura merges with the cervical fascia.

This is the largest organ, and the most pervasive system in the human body: the fascia, which provides the shape and form of the body. Therapists must shift their perspective from looking at a distortion in the skeletal system or in the muscular system, to a distortion that is contained within the fascial system. This is a shift in perspective that therapists must think about, that shape and form are determined by the fascia. Movement is a change in shape of the fascia. That is how movement is defined in this perspective of myofascial release. As one walks, as one crawls, as one sits up, as one runs, an individual perceives movement to be changing continually within the sleeve of various fascial planes. This plastic living tissue is the system that needs to interface myofascial release (Rolf, 1978).

The fascia is multidimensional. It is also an organ of relationship because it forms direct connections with other systems of the body, such as the autonomic nervous system. High sympathetic tone from habituated stress is mediated through the fascial system, because all the connective tissue in the body has sympathetic innervation (Korr, 1979). One can hardly work on soft tissue in the body and not affect the sympathetic nervous system. Myofascial release in particular not only is involved with lengthening and loosening the fascia, which facilitates better movement, but is also involved with lowering sympathetic dominance from habituated stress. The sympathetic nervous system also controls the rate and flow of blood throughout the body. This is called the vasomotor system. When an individual is stressed, the vasomotor system works harder to deliver nutrients to tissue that may also be is chemically compressed from tight fascia. It is important to remember that the sympathetic nervous system innervates all the soft tissue and every blood capillary. The stress of orthopedic injury requires not only myofascial release when indicated, but also input to the sympathetic system to reduce the cycle of steroid secretion. As a secretory system, the sympathetic nervous system often fails to stop producing the irritants even after the initial insult has been dealt with (Willard & Patterson, 1992).

Dropping down to the cellular level of the fascia, cellular biologists have been looking at the fascial system with electron microscopes, and they have discovered that each cell in the body has a connective tissue skeleton called microtubules. At the University of Arizona, microtubules are the subject of some fascinating research on how consciousness is communicated (Freedman, 1994; Horgan, 1994). The shape and form of the cells is also formed by the connective tissue fascia. This is very interesting because the glycoprotein, which is part of the fascial network supporting the cells, extends through the cell membrane, and it connects to a very important component, called the ground substance-extracellular matrix. Cells are connected to the ground substance, and that connection happens as an electrical bonding. The glycoproteins are bathed in a solution of sialic acid. Sialic acid provides an electrical bonding through the ground substance with all the cells in the body (Oschman, 1984). The ground substance is an integral part of the fascial system because it is then connected to the collagen which it surrounds. The key here is that the basis of the tensile strength in the fascia is due to the electrical bonding that occurs at the molecular level of the fascia.

Fascia is an organic crystal. The fascia is a semiconductor. When a crystal is compressed, it generates a weak electrical field called the piezo effect (please refer to the previous chapter). Any kind of movement in the body will compress the fascia. The body has continuous electrical generation in the solid-state circuitry of the fascial system. The body has a flow of electricity generated by the fascial system. This is the realm that one gets into when using manual therapy. A therapist is generating electrical fields via manual compression and active/passive movement, which causes electrical fields in the client to change (Rubik et al., 1994). That electrical current is important because it tells the cells how to pattern their activity.

Some cells are designed to build tissue, and others are designed to help eliminate waste, and so on. This suggests the possibility that some of the problem is in the fascia because its collagen has gotten thick and dense and unable to conduct piezoelectricity through that particular area of the body. Thus the pattern of normal activity is disturbed. This results in shortening and thickening, and a decrease in range of motion.

Electrical conductivity in the tissue is also predicated on the amount of water in the extracellular matrix. This is the ground substance. The ground substance acts like a sponge. Movement and manual therapy changes the hydration of tissue. The other remarkable quality of the ground substance is that it can turn from a solution into a gel and from a gel to a solution, so it is called the gel-sol relationship. The gel-sol relationship occurs when the fascia shortens and thickens, which dehydrates the ground substance. This causes the ground substance to turn from a solution into a gel. Actually, the gel is just like glue. This glue acts as a binder between the various fascial planes and collagen fibers by decreasing the interfiber distance, which allows for collagen to crosslink and increase its tensile strength to protect an area of injury. It produces a restriction of movement, and an extra thickening in the collagen, because the rate of assembly exceeds the rate of removal (Ratner, 1979; Schoenheimer, 1942). The body needs to have rapid adaptive patterning. What that means is that when a person receives an injury—gets bumped, falls, sprains an ankle—the system is designed to build extra tissue around that ankle so that healing can take place. So, please do not break down that tissue until the right healing has taken place.

Collagen is what is worked on in myofascial release. It forms large bundles of fibers called fascia. All the fascial investitures, even the periosteum and the dural membrane that surrounds the brain and spinal cord, the meninges, are made up of collagen. Collagen is an elastic protein. If the right amount of pressure is applied, collagen can be melted and stretched. It has stiffness. The collagen gets stiff when there is a trauma. It has some contractile capability. There is stiffness, elasticity, contractile capability, and tensile strength all in one tough membrane.

When a person begins to increase the palpation skills, he or she begins differentiating the thickness and stiffness in the tissue, which is the collagen density. The tensile strength is very high. Some tissues have the tensile strength of a Goodyear tire—2,000 pounds per square inch (i.e., the dural membrane, the iliotibial [IT] band). The body also has highly developed postural fasciae, like the lumbar fascia and the gluteal fascia (Macintosh, Bogduk, & Gracovetsky, 1987). These are some of the postural fasciae that are important in myofascial release. They get thick; they become undifferentiated; they get very tight and migrate onto other structures. The tendency of the collagen in a stress to the fascial system is to shorten and thicken; it then spreads out with time much like a spider web and continues to decrease movement capability. The dorsal and ventral fasciae of the trunk migrate laterally. Part of the therapist's job is to bring the fascia back toward the midline for better organization.

Tight fascia in a neurologically impaired client is the same as in an orthopedic injury—at the level of the fascia. Movement is restricted. The body continues to build collagen to support the position of the body. The importance is known of movement work with clients to keep their joint spaces open. The experience of feeling stiff and tight is actually extra tissue being built to support position and posture. In myofascial release technique, a therapist is attempting to break this down. The half life of some of these molecules, these building blocks of life, fatty acids and amino acids, is 19 minutes (Schimke & Doyle, 1970). What that means is that the body carries its own quick-drying cement. Say you slump in your chair for an hour listening to a lecture in one of those awful folding metal chairs. A pattern of activity in the collagen has begun to support you by generating cells to build tissue to hold you in this position. It happens that fast. That is why so many clients visit their therapists so often. That is why some of the therapy is so aggressive in order to treat long or severe disability.

Pragmatically, from a therapist's experience of hands-on contact with hypertonic tissue in the over-involved client, that if you take the time and search a muscle that has been hypertonic, what is found are areas within that feel supple and soft—maybe just the size of the pad of the thumbs. What is also found is that there are far more extensive areas where suppleness is lacking, and instead it is rigid, board-like tissue that is not supple and is not spongy. Healthy muscle is 75percent water. The hard thing to imagine, as a therapist, knowing this and working with this for years, is that what is palpating is 75 percent water, and the water is held in a membrane called fascia. When there is neurological or orthopedic involvement, dehydration occurs. Because of mechanical compression, water is driven out of both muscle and fascia. Cardiovascular flow is diminished. Every bundle of muscle fibers has a capillary bed running through it. There are thousands of bundles of muscle fibers in any given long muscle of the body.

The way muscle is designed to work physiologically is contract-relax, contract-relax, contract-relax. What is seen in some types of pathology is bundles of muscle fibers that have been in a contractile state for a period of time. It is just like sucking water through a straw and squeezing that straw, pinching it—the same thing in muscle. The vascular flow is diminished. Muscle is quite unique in that muscle combustion is designed to be aerobic, but it has a backup anaerobic mechanism. This means that even though there is a minimal flow of nutrients and oxygen getting to the tissue, that muscle, when it is neurologically overstimulated, will continue to maintain a spastic state. What ends up is a metabolic wasteland because the muscle is squeezing off the same blood flow that carries off waste products. The primary by-product of muscle combustion, pyruvic acid, cannot enter into the Krebs cycle, cannot be broken down into carbon dioxide and water, and instead ends up as lactic acid and other by-products that accumulate in the muscle and cause what Dr. Janet Travell calls "referred pain" (Travell & Simons, 1998). These by-products are irritants to nerve endings. They cause sensory arousal that will fire back into the cord and will ascend or descend a number of segments and fire out back to other structures whether soft tissue, visceral, cardiovascular, and so on. Each system of the body maps onto the spinal cord differently. An irritated facilitated spinal cord segment(s) will fire back out and cause motor activity that keeps stimulating pain receptors (nociception) elsewhere. For example, if there is involvement in a posterior rotator cuff muscle, the infraspinatus, pain may show up at the base of the skull, in the interscapular space, in the anterior shoulder, elbow, forearm, and/or wrist. That is just one example of somatically referred pain that results from decreased cardiovascular flow. There are also somatic-visceral reflexes that are usually overlooked in a soft tissue practice (Boissonnault & Bass, 1990).

It is hard to believe that once fascia is released it stays that way. Experience reveals that releases are small and tied in to the client's own personal growth, development, and lifestyle. Please remember that the single biggest factor affecting health outcomes in people is their level of education (Pincus & Callahan, 1995). Client education cannot be overlooked either. In many ways, myofascial release is a body education. Therapists are feeding the kinesthetic intelligence of clients (Gardner, 1983). A person's kinesthetic intelligence is located in the myofascia.

CHAPTER 3

Fascia as an Organ of Communication by Robert Schleip

More than 20 years ago, dispute arose between instructors of the Feldenkrais Method of somatic education and teachers of the Rolfing Method of structural integration. Advocates of the second group had claimed that many postural restrictions are because of pure mechanical adhesions and restrictions within the fascial network, whereas the leading figures of the first group suggested that "it's all in the brain," that is, that most restrictions are due to dysfunctions in sensorimotor regulation. They cited a story by Milton Trager, which deals with an old man in a hospital whose body was very stiff and rigid (Trager, Guadagno-Hammond, & Turnley Walker, 1987). But under anesthesia, his muscle tonus got lowered, and he was as limber and soft as a young baby. As soon as his consciousness returned, he got stiff and rigid again.

Subsequently, a small experiment was set up involving several representatives of those two schools, in which three patients underwent an orthopaedic knee surgery. Consent was given to do some passive joint range of motion testing with the three patients before and during anesthesia. With the patient in a supine position, the patient's arms were elevated superiorly above the head and the freedom of movement in this direction was observed. With one of the patients, the elbow dropped all the way to the table above the head before the anesthesia, and this was no different after he lost consciousness.

However, with the other two patients, their elbows could not be elevated all the way in their normal state, that is, their elbows kept hanging somewhere in the air above the head. Five minutes later, when they had lost consciousness, their arms were again elevated above the head, and surprisingly, their elbows dropped all the way down to the table—no restrictions whatsoever, they just dropped! Additionally, the feet of all three patients were dorsiflexed. Here no increased joint mobility during anesthesia could be detected. (Only subjective comparison was used, without any measuring devices.)

The result of the tests was quite shocking. From a Rolfer's point of view, the expectation was that the remaining fascial restrictions would prevent the arms dropping all the way under anesthesia. (The unchanged mobility of the ankle joint was not surprising, because none of the three patients seemed to have any limitations there that would concern a Rolfer.) Given the limited scientific rigor of this preliminary investigation, the result nevertheless convinced that what had been perceived as mechanical tissue fixation may at least be partially due to neuromuscular regulation.

The ongoing interdisciplinary dispute after this event led to a rethinking of traditional concepts of myofascial therapies, and several years later, a first neurologically oriented model was published as a proposed explanatory model for the effects of myofascial manipulation (Cottingham, 1985), later expanded by many others in the field (Schleip, 2003; Figure 3.1).

The body-wide network of fascia is assumed to play an essential role in the posture and movement organization. It is frequently referred to as the organ of form. However for decades, ligaments, joint capsules, and other dense fascial tissues have been regarded as mostly inert tissues and have primarily been considered for their mechanical properties. Nonetheless, in the 1990s, advances were being made in recognizing the proprioceptive nature of ligaments, which subsequently influenced the guidelines for knee and other joint injury surgeries. Similarly, the fascia has been shown

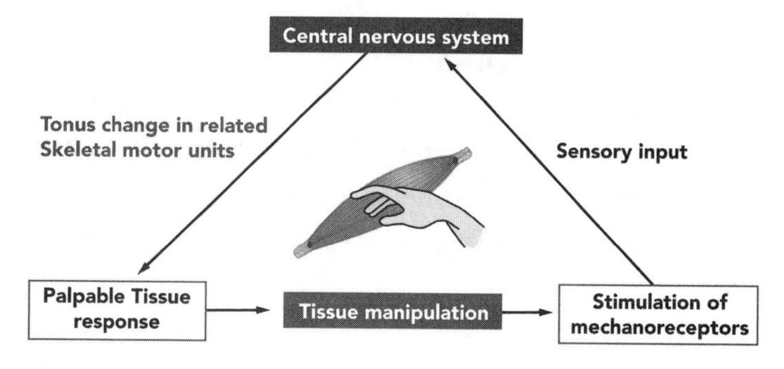

Figure 3.1

to contribute to the sensorimotor regulation of postural control in standing.

It is now recognized that fascial network is one of the richest sensory organs. The surface area of this network is endowed with millions of endomysial sacs and other membranous pockets with a total surface area that by far surpasses that of the skin or any other body tissues. Interestingly, compared with muscular tissue's innervation with muscle spindles, the fascial element of it is innervated by approximately six times as many sensory nerves than its red muscular counterpart. Additionally even the spindle receptors in the muscles are themselves found primarily in areas with force transfer from muscle to connective tissues. This includes many different types of sensory receptors, including the usually myelinated proprioceptive endings such as Golgi, Pacini, and Ruffini endings, but also a myriad of tiny unmyelinated free nerve endings, which are found almost everywhere in fascial tissues, but particularly in periosteum, in endomysial and perimysial layers, and in visceral connective tissues. If these smaller fascial nerve endings are included in the calculation, then the amount of fascial receptors may possibly be equal or even superior to that of the retina, so far considered as the richest sensory human organ. However, for the sensorial relationship with one's own body—whether it consists of pure proprioception, nociception, or the more visceral interoception—fascia provides definitely the most important perceptual organ.

Although fascial stretch therapies and manual fascial therapies often seem to have positive effects on palpatory tissue stiffness, as well as on passive joint mobility, it is still unclear which exact physiological processes may be underlying these responses. Some of the potential mechanisms may be from dynamic changes in water content of the ground substance, altered link proteins in the matrix, or an altered activity of fascial fibroblasts, as well as other factors. However, today an increasing number of practitioners base their concepts to some extent on the mechanosensory nature of the fascial net and its assumed ability to respond to skillful stimulation of its various sensory receptors. The question then is: What is really known about the sensory capacity of fascia? And what specific physiological responses can be expected to elicit in response to stimulation of various fascial receptors?

Fascia has important roles in proprioception, interoception, and nociception. Proprioception is the kinaesthetic sense that enables one to sense the relative position of the parts of the body, posture, balance, and motion. It is usually distinguished from exteroception, which pertains to the stimuli that originate from outside the body, and interoception pertains to how one perceives the sensation related to the physiological needs of the body. Fascial tissues are important for the sense of proprioception (Van der Kolk, 2012). Whereas, in the past, much emphasis was placed on joint receptors (being located in joint capsules and associated ligaments), more recent investigations indicate that more superficially placed mechanoreceptors, particularly in the transitional area between the fascia profunda and the fascia superficialis, seem to be endowed with an exceptionally rich density of proprioceptive nerve endings. Fascia as a network extends throughout the whole body, and numerous muscular expansions maintain it in a basal tension. Thus, it was hypothesized that during a muscular contraction, these expansions could also transmit the effect of the stretch to a specific area of the fascia, stimulating the proprioceptors in that area (Stecco et al., 2007). Although this may be relevant for the practice (and often profound beneficial effects) of skin taping in sports medicine—as well as for other therapeutic fields—further research is necessary to clarify how stimulation of this superficial fascial layer influences proprioceptive regulation in healthy as well as pathological conditions.

A newly rediscovered field is fascial interoception, which relates to mostly subconscious signalling from free nerve endings in the body's viscera—as well as other tissues—informing the brain about the physiological state of the body, and relates it to the need for maintaining homeostasis (Schleip & Jager, 2012). Whereas sensations from proprioceptive receptors are usually projected via their somatomotor cortex, signalling from interoceptive endings is processed via the insula region in the brain and is usually associated with an emotional or motivational component. This field also promises interesting implications for the understanding and treatment of disorders with a somatoemotional component, such as irritable bowel syndrome or essential hypertension.

The sensory nature of fascia includes also its potential for nociception (nociception is the ability to feel pain, caused by stimulation of a nociceptor). Researchers from Heidelberg University (Hoheisel, Taguchi, & Mense, 2012) have conducted research about the nociceptive potential of the lumbar fascia. Their choice of investigating the lumbar fascia is not accidental. Although some cases of lower back pain are definitely caused by deformations of spinal discs, several large magnetic resonance imaging studies clearly reveal that for the majority of lower back pain cases the origin may be elsewhere in the body, as the discal alterations are often purely incidental. Based on this background, a new hypothetical explanation model for lower back pain was proposed by Panjabi (2006) and subsequently elaborated on by others (Langevin & Sherman, 2007; Schleip, Vleeming, Lehmann-Horn, & Klingler, 2007). According to these authors, microinjuries in lumbar connective tissues may lead to nociceptive signalling and further downstream effects associated with lower back pain. The new findings from the Heidelberg group show the nociceptive potential of the lumbar fascia; in patients with nonspecific lower back pain, their fascial tissue maybe a more important pain source than the lower back muscles or other soft tissues. The findings have potentially huge implications for the diagnosis and treatment of lower back pain. As this is a newly emerging field, their research will definitely trigger further research investigations into this important field within modern health care.

These exciting new topics from research might lead to new insights to clinical applications. They are fully discussed in the book *Fascia: The Tensional Network of the Human Body: The Science and Clinical Applications in Manual and Movement Therapy.* (Edited By Robert Schleip, Thomas W. Findley, Leon Chaitow, Peter A. Huijing. Published by Elsevier. See www.tensionalnetwork.com for more information.)

Robert Schleip, Ph.D., is an international Rolfing instructor and fascial anatomy teacher. Robert has been an enthusiastic certified Rolfer since 1978. He holds an M.A. degree in psychology, and he is a certified Feldenkrais teacher since 1988. He earned his Ph.D. with honors in 2006, established the Fascia Research Project at Ulm University shortly thereafter, and presently has a lab of his own. He was coinitiator and organizer of the first Fascia Research Congress at Harvard Medical School in Boston in 2007.

CHAPTER 4

The Skills of Myofascial Release

Myofascial release requires more skill than knowledge. The skills of touching another person's body are of paramount importance in a therapeutic relationship. For the sake of simplicity, a set of four categories of skills are devised to reveal what is foundational to the application of the myofascial release technique. These four areas of skill are called contact, sensing, verbal, and action skills. Look briefly at each one of them and learn what they consist of.

Contact Skills

> *To be in contact, one needs to be grounded, have adequate boundaries, enjoy unrestricted breathing, have access to feeling, and have the intention to be present. To be fully present reflects a functional and durable sense of self.*
> (Conger, 1994, p. 56)

1. The first contact skill is the ability to relate to your own respiratory pattern. "How are you breathing?" "Can you connect with your breath while in contact with the client?" Your breathing tells you a lot about your inner state, and the respiratory diaphragm is the fulcrum around which the entire myofascial system is oriented. What this means is to begin paying attention to your own body and physiology to access information about the client.

2. Whenever you apply compressional force into the client's tissues, you must maintain an awareness of length in your spine. As you make contact with the client, sense your own spine and begin to stretch and lengthen, especially through the joints of your wrists, arms, and neck. In addition, you want to move your head and spine away from and in opposition to the vector of force that you are using to enter the tissues.

3. Maintain an awareness of where your feet are on the ground while you are working. You do not want to position your feet too far lateral or too far back of each other. You might even want to play with positioning yourself to get a slight stretch into your hamstrings to prevent your spine from becoming kyphotic as you apply pressure into the client. Generally speaking, you want to keep your shoulder girdle and pelvic girdle in a perpendicular alignment to the line of force or vector that you are applying into the client.

4. Centering is a technique that involves paying attention to any sensations that arise in your body while you are working. Sensations can arise in your low back or in your legs, maybe in your chest or just about anywhere. Rather than discard and ignore these sensations, you want to become curious about them and bring awareness to them.

5. You want to have a relationship with your mind and thoughts that come up during a session. You especially want to resist impulses to fix the client. Try and maintain neutrality and curiosity rather than a more aggressive position of trying to fix or eliminate the client's symptoms.

Sensing

1. Sensing requires some practice. Therapists tend to enter tissue much too quickly. Sensing is the first method you will use to begin gathering useful information about the client, as well as his or her tissues.

2. Sensing comes from a place of neutrality. If you try placing gentle buoyant hands somewhere on the body and you are receptive to the motility of the tissues, you can then begin to sense an ease in the tissue movement or a lack of movement. Serge Paoletti describes it this way, "When the hand is placed on the tissues, you should get an impression of floating in all spatial planes, as if your hand were resting on a soft surface which is floating on a basin filled with water" (Paoletti, 2006, p. 207). Paoletti calls this listening.

3. If you think you felt something, you felt it. Try to keep your intentions spontaneous rather than narrow focused. If you work from a place of openness and curiosity, then anything can happen.

4. See if you can connect on a heart level with clients. What that means is bring awareness to your heart. Soften it. See if you can go one step further and sense the client's heart from a place in your own heart. What you are doing is working from a place of love rather than a place of judgment. That means putting all preconceived ideas away and starting from scratch. It will take some practice, but it is worth the effort. Research shows that the tissues will respond when the connection is more harmonious.

Verbal

1. The most important verbal command is the Rule of Stop. Clients need to be given permission to say stop. It isn't something that comes naturally for some people. Some clients will feel that they will be hurting the therapist's feelings if they ask to stop. The client needs to be verbally empowered to tell the therapist when to stop, when to slow down, and when to back off. It is extremely important to take the time to sit the client down and create a contract between the two of you. This contract can be part of your informed consent. Let them know that you need them to tell you to stop if something is uncomfortable. A therapist can be working on a client who appears relaxed, when in fact the client could be in full terror mode. Use your soft seeing skills and check in. This is crucial because of the potential to drive trauma deeper.

2. For manual therapy to be effective, a client needs to be coached to be able to bring his or her awareness into the tissue, right where the therapist is working. This too can be hard for some clients, but it is a big part of the job and a big part of healing just to be present in the body. This presence needs to facilitate both through modalities and education. Therapists are trying to have people reconnect with their pain. They need breath to facilitate a release, not only for emotional pain, but also the physical pain.

3. Listening to both verbal and nonverbal aspects of the client's story is a primary skill in a holistic practice of myofascial release. Failure to listen carefully and sensitively leads a therapist to make judgments that are academic and lack subjective understanding of a unique story each client brings to the treatment room.

4 A client's body can inform a therapist about many things that can only be found out by listening to the client's words.

5. Appreciate the uniqueness of the whole client by carefully listening and observing.

6. Refer out when necessary.

Action

1. The hallmark of this direct work, Ida Rolf use to say, is to enter the tissue mindfully, find what is tight, take the tissue to its restriction barrier, and move the tissue into its anatomically correct position while asking for movement. The tightness might have one direction of tightness or it might be tight in more than one direction.

2. Apply direct pressure with several pounds of pressure and sometimes even 15 to 20 pounds of pressure over a given area of the body. It might be over a bone or tendon, too. Remember that each client is unique, with his or her own story and his or her own body type. The older the adhesions, the more effort it will take to make a difference.

3. The sooner a therapist can work the tissues following any kind of injury or trauma, the better the outcome.

4. Move slowly into the tissues at all times. There are no exceptions to this rule. Greet the tissue with mindful hands, sink gently, and move slowly.

5. Allow the client to verbally direct the pressure at any time by saying "slow down," "stop right there just for a second," or "lighten up for just a minute."

6. Use soft seeing skills at all times. You want to keep your eyes open and continually scan the client's body looking for defensive physiology.

7. Ask the client for movements occasionally that serve two purposes. It distracts the client for a time, but more important than that, it facilitates the fascia to release. The movements that you ask for need to be done slowly.

8. Continue to direct the client to take deep breaths into the area that you are working. This is probably the best skill to remember. This is the most effective way to integrate the work into the nervous system.

9. Watch always for activation of the autonomic nervous system and apply the skills necessary. Recognition of the sympathetic nervous system is clinically important, as overexcitement of the sympathetic nervous system leads to hyperarousal and greatly diminishes the effectiveness of holistic myofascial release.

10. Be mindful of your own body mechanics and remember that you as the therapist must take time for self care.

CHAPTER 5

Treatment Strategies

The Therapeutic Relationship

The session begins when the client calls the clinic and makes the appointment. A therapist takes this time to ask any important health history questions. "Is there anything that needs to be known about the client's physical or emotional health before the appointment?" "What is the client's goal for the session?" This will give you time to prepare and be ready when the client walks in the door. Once the client comes through the front door and you greet her warmly, many things are happening. The client is wondering if she is going to like you. She may be wondering if this is a safe place to be. You can convey a sense of safety and a sense of trust right in the moment by making eye contact, being genuine, warm, and connecting at a heart level. This is all part of forming the therapeutic container or relationship. The health history and informed consent are also a very important part of this process. Full disclosure between the client and therapist makes for a safe and effective treatment between the therapist and the client.

Presence and attention on the part of the therapist is important. One must wake up those senses and become aware of his or her own body sensations in this healing journey with the client. Research shows that "the quality of the therapeutic relationship is based on ethical behavior, clear boundaries, and the therapist's own body and mind. This quality of attention influences the nervous system of the client" (Bechara & Naqvi, 2004). The bottom line is it is not the technique so much as the relationship that is formed with the client that matters the most. It is about client-centered care, but it is also about the therapist and his or her role in serving others.

The therapeutic relationship involves the most appropriate use of the therapist's knowledge, skills, and abilities to help serve the goals of the client. Although it is sometimes implied that therapists must be free of their own agendas for the session, therapists and clients must discuss and agree upon a shared intention or goal for the treatment plan. Shared goals must be realistic and clear. The return to health takes longer than most clients imagine. It is important that these shared goals are not exclusively dictated by the therapist but are created in conjunction with the client. Shared goals between the client and therapist must include trust, expected outcomes, appropriate boundaries, and most of all, safety.

Empathy

Empathy is the ability to sense the feelings and emotions of another person. Discreet parts of the therapist's brain actually sense the client's feelings and emotions by observing the vocal tone, facial expression, and body movement of the client. This is done by a set of what are called mirror neurons, which exist in the brain and heart of every human being. Once the feelings of another person are mirrored in a brain and heart, they are sensed through the body of the recipient (or therapist in this context). This quality of mirroring is frequently unconscious, and it is the responsibility of the therapist to become aware of his or her own body, especially when working with a client. Body awareness can be cultivated through various skills, from yoga to meditation. Therapists can thus make a distinction between their own feelings and emotions and those of the clients. This conscious attention to body sensation builds resonance and safety for the client (Siegel, 1999). Resonance is the neurological phenomenon of one's nervous system being able to synchronize with another nervous system.

As this process of resonance emerges, empathy is deepened into compassion, which is simply knowing what to do next for the client. It is enhanced in such a way that the client naturally feels safe, by sensing the empathy of the therapist. The therapist, likewise, can also sense the client's increasing sense of safety. It is like a circuit between two people; each reinforcing and enhancing empathy in each other. This is called interpersonal neurobiology (IPNB) in the scientific literature (Siegel, 2010). Each person in the therapeutic relationship knows the other is being held with the intention of empathy and compassion. This ultimately promotes relaxation and ultimately an environment for healing.

There is a big difference between sympathy and empathy. Sympathy is like a one-way street in which one person can think about the experience of another person with heart-centered caring. This is not the same as feeling what the other person feels.

Empathy has been linked to oxytocin, the hormone associated with the felt sense of love in a relationship. The deepest level of nurturing, called love, can actually take place during a treatment session. Love is the feeling of being deeply supported and cared for. When one first cultivates empathy and compassion with body awareness, love automatically manifests. This can be enhanced by the simple habit of the therapist taking time to periodically cultivate thoughts and feelings of loving kindness. Loving kindness starts with regularly declaring gratitude for people and events in one's life. It is as simple as sensing the movement of the heartbeat in the middle of one's chest. This is known to enhance empathy and, thus, loving kindness toward others.

Tips on Proper Execution

Proper execution is the practice of mindful hands that land softly, work slowly, and pause occasionally. The therapist looks and lands gently, searching subtly. One does not poke, shove, or push around in the tissue. When in doubt, just rest a hand gently on the tissue and follow the client's breathing.

1. Take the time to position your body for maximum ease and strength, staying as perpendicular to the contact as possible. Keep your own pelvis and shoulder girdle in alignment with your direction of force.

2. Find the stuck layer by moving in slowly at a 90-degree angle. Imagine your contact is a curved line as you do this.

3. Once you find the layer you want, change your angle gradually, applying a gliding pressure to the stuck layer at an oblique angle. Move where the tissue remains stuck (hard, nonmobile). Again, think of a mobile, dynamic, curved line as you do this, as though your contact was a snake slithering in liquid tissue.

4. Make small, rolling, sliding micromovements into the stuck areas or along the edge of hardened tissue. In general, try to move tissue into its anatomically correct position by moving though restriction barriers. This is direct technique.

5. Then ask for movement at the position to amplify sensation or to engage the stuck layer. Asking for breath increases awareness and decreases intense sensation. It integrates the nervous system with the myofascia. Be curious about the cause of the stuckness.

6. A liquid softening or buoyancy will occur in the area where you are working. Stop at that point. This signifies a release. Analyze where to go next and then move on.

Sometimes you will get an autonomic cue that a release has occurred, like a deep breath rather than a tissue sensation or heat.

7. Do not spend more than a minute or so in one placement. If nothing is happening, move somewhere else. (Though it may only be 1/2 inch away or less.)

8. Work on and around bony margins, as the deep and superficial fascia merge there. Remember that bone is considered soft tissue in this work.

9. Visualize the anatomical structures underneath your touch and intend to connect with them through the fascia, their covering.

10. Releases occur in many different ways, not just in the tissue. Do not restrict your awareness to the tissue dynamics. Remember, if you think you felt it move, you felt it. The human hand is capable of perceiving a movement one one-hundredth the width of a human hair.

Alternately, keep your feet together under your pelvis rather than one foot way in front of the other. This will save wear and tear on your spine.

Tips on Asking for Movement

Asking for gentle movement helps engage the tissue with which is being worked. It helps the therapist to sense the line of restriction in the connective tissue. It maintains the verbal interaction between the therapist and the client, and can decrease the sense of discomfort for the client. A therapist must be sure the client is able to isolate only the movement the therapist has requested and keep scanning the client to be sure he or she is not moving unnecessarily.

1. Stand the client up at the beginning and end of each session and ask her to walk. It gives you a whole different view than just looking at her statically. Try standing the client up periodically during the session, as well.

2. Ask for movement prior to beginning contact to observe where the connective tissue is immobile or where the movement may appear to be out of proportion.

3. When working, ask for small movements after you have found the restriction. Start with an inch and ask for more or less as needed. Look for the first engagement of the movement. Large or gross motor movement is superficial and overrides the deep fascia. Tell the client you just want to see the first inch of movement, then say give me half of that, and so on.

4. At first, the client will tend to give you too large and too fast a movement. She will need to be educated to give you just far enough and slow enough to engage the layer being worked.

5. Ask for one movement at a time until you have found the right one. That opens the tissue to change.

6. Ask the client to move into your hands. Don't keep digging when the client relaxes.

7. Movement you can ask for:

- Breathe—particularly into the point of contact. Then breathe out—letting go of the sensation.

- Move into me, from the inside, or let your bone come toward me, or move just this disc. Movements that clients do not know, or at best are difficult to do, will cause consciousness to move into the deep fascia. Just think about trying to move a disc!

- Ask for movement at the proximal joint to where you are working. Ask for movement that you know will engage the muscle group surrounding the area where you are working.

- Have the client go through a full, slow range of movement if increased range of motion is one of your goals.

8. Until you are comfortable with these skills, do not ask for more than one movement at a time. Gradually during the session you can ask for multiple sequential movements.

9. Cue the client's breath with one or both of your hands. Place a hand on an area you plan to work on or have just worked on and ask for a breath into that area. When it is convenient, place one hand in front and one hand in back of the body and slowly direct the client's breath between your two hands before or after contact. Ask for a slow, easy breath that moves up and down the front of the spine.

10. While working most anywhere, you can ask the client to occasionally move her tailbone. This will access the deeper fascia around the psoas muscle.

11. Have the client visualize the organ or area you are working on. Show her an image from an anatomy book. Ask her to direct her breath around and into that area. Ask her to imagine she can move the organ. This accesses other parts of the brain and will help integrate the work.

Avoiding Autonomic Exhaustion

Discharge from the autonomic nervous system can result from this work. It is noted by flushing of the skin, sweating and clamminess, fasciculation, and sometimes emotional release. Autonomic activation during this work cannot be avoided. However, the intensity of the discharge following the activation can be moderated by employing the following techniques:

1 Pace the work you are doing. Allow the client the time to connect with each maneuver and time, between each maneuver, to "settle back down." Allow for two or three cycles of respiration every couple of minutes without your hand on the client. Scan the whole body continually.

2. Stay in verbal contact with the client by asking, "How are you feeling?," "Are you doing OK?," or "Am I moving too fast?" Then listen to her voice or observe her body for cues.

3. Watch the client's eyes and skin color. Watch for clamminess or fasciculation that is shaking or tremoring in the extremities. If you notice signs of autonomic activation or discharge, slow down and quiet down your work. Occasionally place your hands on or around her diaphragm and just listen for several minutes.

4. An occasional deep breath can decrease autonomic discharge. Do not overdo this however. Avoid hyperventilation. Tell the client to slow her breath. You can put your hand over her diaphragm for a minute or so to calm them down.

5. You can see where autonomic excitement is not happening. It is best to have autonomic discharge occurring throughout the body. Autonomic engagement will

generally be inhibited at one of the major transverse diaphragms—the A-0 joint, thoracic, respiratory, or pelvic diaphragms. Keep these diaphragms open and released during your work. Gentle encouragement on the back of the neck, costal arch, or belly is often enough to open a diaphragm. You can also add a verbal cue, such as, "Can you let that feeling you are having in your chest come down to your leg," "Can you allow the shaking in your leg to move into your belly," and so on. Just ask the client to connect the area that is shaking to the next closest one that is not.

6. Allow the client to shake off or shudder off the energy that has built up. This is a vagotonic response and looks different than a sympathetic discharge. The spine will arch, and it will happen in a wave-like pattern every couple of minutes during a discharge cycle. This is parasympathetic tone rising. Headaches and nausea are also vagal responses that are strong.

7. Moving too fast into traumatized tissue or into a jerk or tickle response area can lead to autonomic spikes. You can drive trauma deeper as well, so slow down. Driving the trauma deeper means that the organs along with their fascia can contract, or the autonomic system can dissociate.

8. If a client has had some autonomic discharge during a session, let her rest quietly before getting up and have her move about slowly until she gets her bearings. Be sure she is breathing normally. You can direct her breathing and ask her to take long slow breaths, especially into her abdomen, pelvis, and upper ribs.

9. Ask the client to allow the movement, shaking, or trembling deeper into her organs. Name an organ for her.

Sometimes you can direct this energy into her bones or other systems that might be stuck (i.e., kidney problem, ulcer, constipation). "Can you let the trembling into your liver," and "Can you let the shaking into your bones?" This allows for a much deeper integration into the nervous system.

10. Your job is to guide the sympathetic system discharge and then assist the client in containing the charge in the viscera, the parasympathetic system, while she reorganizes and renegotiates the trauma.

These are the elements of soft seeing. Manual therapy has evolved from just working with tissue release to larger systemic issues with the autonomic nervous system. It is important to be able to facilitate the discharge patterns inherent in the autonomic nervous system to affect a greater integration of the client's reporting systems and history.

Support During Emotional Release

It is not uncommon for a client to express emotion within the context of a myofascial release session. Working deep in the body may trigger a cascade of chemicals that results in an emotional release. Unless a therapist is a licensed mental health care worker, processing these emotions is beyond the scope of practice and is unethical. On the other hand, empathy and compassion are appropriate responses as the therapist assists the client. Below are some tips for managing emotional release.

- Offer tissues if the client is crying
- Ask gently, "How may I help you?," "What do you need right now?," or "Would you like to end the session?"

- Be present and stay in the moment with the client, listening with an open heart
- Remember, the therapist does not need to do anything
- Keep breathing and remain centered and grounded
- Encourage the client to keep breathing
- Facilitate grounding for the client by asking permission to touch the feet
- Allow time for quiet, if needed
- Allow time for talking, if needed
- Use reflective listening when appropriate by nodding the head up and down, with sounds of acknowledgement
- Be supportive and accepting
- Maintain a safe space for the client
- Respect what has happened, and remember this may be a very important event in the client's life
- Refrain from giving advice
- Refrain from withdrawal, judgment, and using psychotherapeutic techniques
- Own your personal feelings; honestly acknowledge and take responsibility for how you are feeling (to yourself)

It is very common for the therapist to have personal issues triggered by a client who is also triggered. In the long term, therapists need to increase their own self-awareness and work to become more comfortable when the client's feelings are elicited. Taking this event to a supervisor for help could be very valuable. Therapists need to learn to temporarily put aside their own issues during a session, until after the client has left, and seek appropriate help if necessary. The massage therapist must avoid processing psychological material. This work falls within the domain of psychotherapy. The following must be avoided by the therapist for ethical practice:

- Eliciting or encouraging the client to give more information about an event by asking "What happened after that?" or "What did you do then?"
- Encouraging stronger emotional release
- Suggesting what the emotional material might be related to
- Focusing on emotional problems
- Interpreting either verbal information or emotional expression

CHAPTER 6

The Myofascial Release Session

Warm up Superficially

With the client lying in a prone position take a moment or two to ground. You can place gentle hands on the client's sacrum and heart, or sacrum and C7. Allow yourself to connect with the client's breath and accommodate the breath as it comes into your hands. If you are not feeling breath in both of your hands, encourage the client verbally to see if she can find your hands with her breath. You may want to cycle through two or three respirations before slowly taking your hands away. Another opportunity for connecting or beginning a session is to assist the client in doing a brief body scan. For example, you might ask her to bring her awareness into the treatment room. Maybe cue her to hear the gentle running of the hydrocolator or the music playing. Then ask her to bring her awareness to her body, particularly the surface of her skin. "How does your skin feel as it's making contact with the sheets?" Ask her to bring awareness to her feet, her legs, and her pelvis. Continue through her belly, chest, arms, neck, and face. Remind her that she has a front, a back, and even side bodies. Why is this important? It is important because healing takes place inside the body. People live outside of their bodies. Sometimes it is scary for an individual to come into relationship with their own body. It can feel uncomfortable for some people. Practicing body scans slows down a stressed out body. Sometimes coaching the client to just place her own hand over her heart and deep breathe is enough. It gives the client a secure and safe internal base. For example, if you have somebody come in, and she is stressed out and has had a hard day already—especially for those folks that like to come in at the end of the day—do some breath work with her. You could begin just checking the individual ribs. Clients look forward to this time in a session as a way of orienting to the present moment, and they learn to use it as a resource daily in their own lives as a mindful meditation.

Finding the right pacing for each unique client is necessary. Using the breath or a brief body scan is a good start to the session. This is where you begin to test the client's autonomic flexibility before going into the deep fascias.

It is always a safe idea to begin the session on the superficial fascias over the erectors and back. This is a neutral place, unlike starting the client supine, which is a much more vulnerable position. Another option is to work on the lower extremities. It is an osteopathic model. It is also a Rolfing model. That model is to start at the feet and work up. Think about lifting the ventral fasciae up the front and dropping it over the shoulders and down the back. This creates a stable base to build upon. The neurodevelopmental therapy model says that the trunk is actually the base. Look at the different approaches, listen to your gut, and see what works best for the clients. The bottom line is keeping the idea of wholeness as you do your work. The body is not just a shoulder, not just a knee. Everything is connected through this fascial system, and it needs to be treated as the whole organism that it is.

Go Deeper

There is the potential of driving one's trauma deeper if you work too fast or without permission. Remember to reinforce the Rule of Stop. Keep your eyes open. Scan the body watching for autonomic discharge. The more stressed out a body is, the slower you need to work. Pull out 3 to 5 releases in one session. If you are working a 60-minute session, work superficially for the first 20 to 30 minutes, work deep tissue for 20 to 30 minutes, and close with integration techniques. In a 90-minute session, work deep tissue for approximately 45 minutes. Of course you would not hesitate to shorten that time if the client becomes activated or overstimulated. Look for the window of ease into the system. It does not serve the client to wait until the last 15 minutes to pull out a psoas release or to decide to work on the adductors. If she asks for more, gently explain why this would not be an appropriate choice. This will shift the session into an integrative mode and help to wrap up the session.

You must negotiate a verbal contract with the client. It is important in all areas of bodywork but especially when doing deep tissue. It can even be part of your written informed consent. The verbal contract might include things like "We are going to monitor your pain levels by working within a pain scale. Zero is no pain and 10 is like slamming your finger in a car door. We don't want to work at a pain level greater than a 7 or 8. Please let me know and I can either lighten or deepen my pressure." You might explain to her that the pain that you feel is a "hurt so good pain" or a pain that is like a deep itch finally being satisfied. There should be no splinting or activation of the sympathetic nervous system. Enter the tissue mindfully. You can find appropriate pressure by setting down lightly, enter and sink slowly, and then move once you feel a softening. There are many things to be aware of when working the deeper fasciae.

You need to be monitoring the quality, quantity, depth, duration, and direction each moment. This means staying in the present moment yourself. This is how you help the client integrate her experience. This autonomic discharge becomes an option and not a necessity. What is too much and what is too little in regards to your touch? Where are the client's resources located in her body? How can you best support the client's inherent resources? Where is she strong in her body? Make your touch slow and incremental.

In chemistry, this is called titration. As you work the tissue slowly and mindfully, there may be a moment of critical mass when some kind of transformation occurs morphologically and systemically. When you titrate your input, this allows the client to utilize the bioelectrical magnetic energy that is freed up. You will decrease the chance of overloading her nervous system (Levine, 2010).

Refer back to Chapter 1 for a more in-depth discussion about treatment possibilities like the triad model, organizational concepts, and disengagement. In addition, throughout the manual, there are numerous reminder boxes to help you organize a safe and effective treatment plan.

Integration

After you have done some deep fascial intervention, then you want to work the integrative fasciae to finish the session. Things like sacral balancing techniques are lovely to end the session with. In addition, the atlanto-occipital joint release or working the suboccipitals, temporalis, and the fasciae of the head feel exquisite. Bring your work back to the head, spine, and sacrum. Bring your work back to the midline of the body and connect the midline from top to bottom and bottom to top. Long effleurage strokes that run slowly from the head to the foot and the foot to the head bring a sense of wholeness and completeness to the session.

Reeducation

The last part of this process is reeducation. Everyone has a different way of working with reeducation. If you have been trained in neurodevelopmental therapy, you are going to do movement work. You might show clients some stretching and various exercises. Yoga classes are a great thing to recommend. In addition, have your contact list filled with appropriate referrals like a good nutritionist, counselor, colonics specialist, or physical therapist for example. It is always good practice to know when to refer out.

CHAPTER 7

Indications and Contraindications for Myofascial Release

The biggest contraindication for the application of any manual therapy is whether it is personally felt to be safe, regardless of what condition the client is reporting. Safety is a subjective factor in which a therapist must simply listen to his or her own mind, and if the therapist has any doubts whether myofascial release would be effective at this particular moment, the therapist must not do it. That being said, there are, of course, numerous indications such as these listed below and followed by the traditional contraindications.

Indications

Ankle

Achilles tendinitis
Flexor tendinitis
Plantar fascitis
Tarsal tunnel syndrome
Pes cavus (claw foot)
Inversion sprain
Ligament sprain: Calcaneofibular, Ant. talofibular, Post talofibular, Talonavicular

Knee

Chondromalacia of patella
Patellarfemoral dysfunction
Patellar tendinitis
Medial/lateral collateral ligament sprain
Pes anserinus tendinitis—three insertions: sartorius, gracilis, semitendinosus
Bursitis: Infrapatellar, suprapatellar, and so on (There are nineteen bursae around the knee.)
Total knee replacement

Hip and Thigh

Trochanteric bursitis
Meralgia paresthetica (outer thigh)
IT band syndrome
Piriformis syndrome
Psoas dysfunction
Gluteal tendinitis
Adductor tendinitis
Chronic hip displacement
Total hip replacement
Ligament sprain: iliofemoral, pubofemoral, ischiofemoral

Low Back and Hip

Lumbar strain
Lumbar dysfunction
Lumbar spondylosis
Sciatica
Lumbosacral radiculitis
Sacroiliac instability
Sacral sprain
Coccygodynia (pain)
Vertebral fusion

Laminectomy
Spinal stenosis scoliosis
Ankylosing spondylitis

Neck

Traumatic cervical sprain
Spasmodic torticollis
Brachial radiculitis
Cephalgia
Thoracic outlet syndrome
Cervical stenosis

Shoulder

Adhesive shoulder capsulitis
Rotator cuff syndrome
Supraspinatus syndrome
Biceps tendinitis
Chronic dislocations
Ligament sprain: acromioclavicular, coracoclavicular, coracoacromial; coracohumeral, glenohumeral, transverse humeral, medial deltoid
Bursitis: subacromial, subcoracoid, subdeltoid

Wrist and Hand

Carpal tunnel syndrome
Palmar fasciitis
Tendinitis of hand or wrist
Tunnel syndromes

Cranial Region

TMJ dysfunction
Tinnitus
Sinusitis
Tension headaches

Systemic Musculoskeletal

Angina pectoris
Palindromic rheumatism
Arthritis (25 different types)
Calcification of joint
Fibromyositis
Progressive myositis ossificans
Neuralgia, neuritis
Dysmenorrhea

Systemic Nervous

Bell's palsy
Horner's syndrome
Neuropathy; entrapment
Paresthesia
Tic douloureux
Trigeminal neuralgia
Spastic cerebral palsy
Spasticity due to stroke

Contraindications

One of the first things that you learn in massage school is to first do no harm. This list may not include a particular contraindication that relates to the client's health history. Creating a treatment plan and taking the time to thoroughly assess the client will ensure the safety of the client.

Acute circulatory conditions

Acute rheumatoid arthritis

Acute trauma/inflammation

Advanced degenerative changes

Advanced diabetes

Aneurysm

Anticoagulant therapies

Cellulitis

Colds and flu

Contagious skin conditions

Decreased sensation/neuropathy

Extreme pain

Febrile state (fever)

Fibromyalgia

Healing fractures

Hypersensitivity of skin

Malignancy

Obstructive edema

Open wounds

Osteomyelitis

Osteoporosis

Structural issues

Systemic or localized infections

Sutures

SECTION 2

Photographic Atlas

CHAPTER 8

Releases of the Spine and Thorax

Functional Breath Releases

Very often clients will exhibit a pattern of a rigid or frozen rib cage from shock or trauma. The underlying respiratory pattern is either very rapid, which leads toward hyperventilation, or very slow, leading toward hypoventilation. These patterns in turn lead to what is called respiratory acidosis, meaning there are elevated levels of carbon dioxide in the system or respiratory alkalosis with elevated levels of oxygen in the bloodstream. For whatever the reason, the ribs are stuck, and therefore, the whole bony trunk is fixated. This appears outwardly as though someone is barrel-chested, or the opposite pattern, which is one of depression. Depression here is the sense that the rib cage is moved inferiorly, thus pulling the head forward and contributing to what is called forward head posture. The first thing that happens in any orthopedic or neurological trauma is called the startle reflex mechanism. This startle reflex mechanism is a very quick inhalation in order to fix the upper ribs on inhalation to ensure that the thoracic outlet stays open. Soft tissue management of orthopedic injuries and other types of traumas very often overlook the underlying respiratory pattern once the manipulation has been completed. These techniques are designed to open up the rib cage and create a fuller range of motion during breathing and, in general, to mobilize the enormous amount of joint spaces in the trunk. It is important to bear in mind that the number one intention of these releases is to focus on the breath and not on the soft tissue or bones. This work requires concentration on the therapist's part, and coordination between his or her palpation skills, amount of pressure, and verbal skills. Those verbal skills are soliciting an in-breath and an out-breath along with the pressure being used. Finally, use the visual skills to keep scanning the trunk while applying these techniques, which will help determine their effectiveness. The four functional breath releases are accomplished in the following manner.

Functional Breath Release One

Begin by compressing gently on the rib cage while the client is exhaling. While compressing the rib cage, motion test the ribs and trunk in the three different vectors or directions. They are medial toward the spine, inferiorly toward the pelvis, and posteriorly toward the table, assuming that the client is in supine position. Make the evaluation of which vector or direction is the most fixated while you are following the client's first or second cycle of exhalation. Decide which vector needs to be reinforced, and on the third and fourth cycles of exhalation, compress the rib cage in that one direction only. Make sure you have completely caused the client to exhale both mechanically with your pressure, which can be upward to 20 or 30 pounds of pressure, as well as verbally, asking the client to exhale even more when you feel you are at the end point of her excursion. Remove your pressure in each of the preceding steps while the client inhales. Do not completely remove your hands, but do not restrict her ability to inhale. This step also includes more verbal contact because you need to direct the client to breathe in when you have also asked her to exhale more fully.

Figure 8.1 shows the therapist's hands on the right side of the rib cage with the left hand placed firmly over the pectoral area and the right hand on the costal arch and above. It is important not to compress the breast as this is not only uncomfortable, but unnecessary.

With both hands on the right side of the rib cage, apply the steps as listed above. Follow the client's breathing for one or two cycles with a very light pressure just getting a sense of her breathing. You will find as you work these techniques, that often just in following the client's breath with no pressure, you will get a sense of which direction is more stuck. This is a good example of sensing. Once you have followed her breath for a little bit, instruct the client to take a deep breath and at the peak of that deep breath, say "slowly exhale and let all the air out" and coordinate the pressure with her exhalation and slowly start to compress the rib cage. For a few seconds press medially, and on the same exhalation for a few seconds press inferiorly toward the pelvis, and for a few more seconds press the rib cage posteriorly. Although the posterior compression requires you to shift the position of your hands slightly toward the anterior part of the rib cage, it is no problem to shift your hands while doing this technique. It is also important that the application of this technique be done on the coronal plane of the body and that the pressure is started evenly with both hands. Very often the client will report she feels more pressure on one hand than the other.

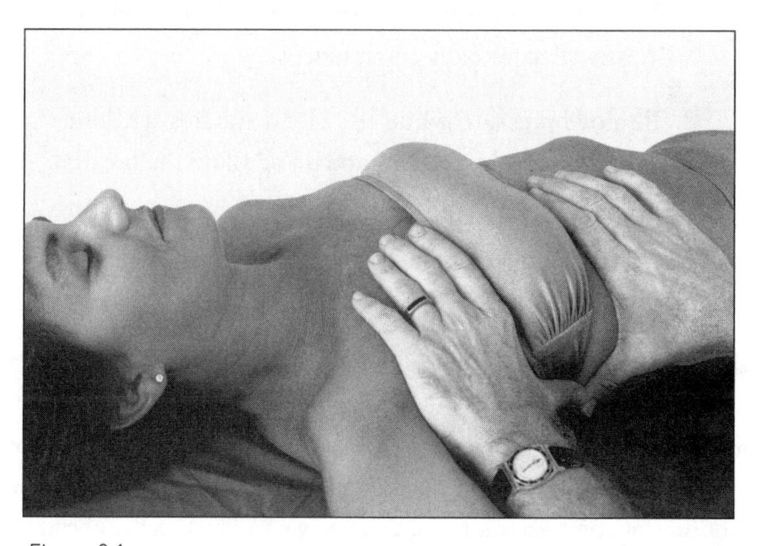

Figure 8.1

The Work: Breath Release One

Client Position: Supine

1. Begin with one hand over the pectorals and the other hand over the costal arch.

2. With light touch, monitor or listen to the client's breathing.

3. Compress the ribcage while the client is exhaling.

4. While compressing the ribcage, in a single exhale, motion-test the ribs and trunk in three different vectors: toward the spine, toward the pelvis/feet, toward the table.

5. Make an evaluation of the vector that is most stuck following cycles of exhalation.

6. Decide which vector needs to be reinforced, and on the third and fourth cycles of exhalation, compress the ribcage in that one direction only.

7. Make sure the client has exhaled completely; mechanically, as well as verbally cuing her.

8. Remove pressure while the client inhales without removing hands. Just accommodate or allow the breath while keeping contact.

Functional Breath Release Two

The second technique begins with one hand over the length of the sternum of the client with the heel of your hand on the manubrium and fingertips over the xiphoid process. In this position, you can really only check two vectors; posterior compression toward the table and inferior compression toward the pelvis. Your other hand can be placed over your working hand for support as shown in Figure 8.2. Sense which motion is most restricted and place your emphasis on the restriction.

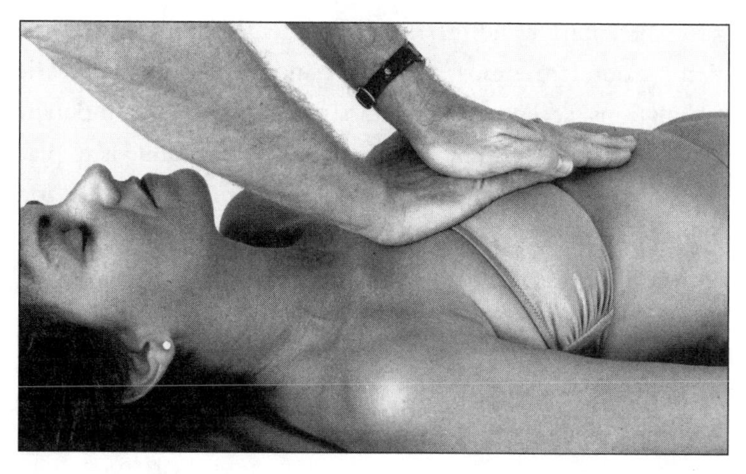

Figure 8.2

The Work: Breath Release Two

Client Position: Supine

1. Begin with one hand over the length of the sternum, with the heel of the hand on the manubrium and the fingertips over the xiphoid process. Your other hand is used for support.

2. The vectors are toward the table and toward the pelvis.

3. Judge the motion that is most restricted and place emphasis on the restriction.

Functional Breath Release Three

The third technique begins with the client in prone position with your hands over the scapula and rib cage, shown in Figure 8.3. It is important to not compress the spine as part of this technique, but to stay focused on the scapula and rib cage. Once again, start by coming to neutral with your hands. Follow the client's breath, and compress as she exhales. In this case you are just motion testing for the anterior and inferior component of her breath. Sense which motion is the most restricted, and on the next two series of exhalations, accentuate that missing or restricted component. One important thing to remember with this technique is to place a pillow under the client, especially if they are female. You don't have to particularly compress the scapula either in this case if the client can hang her arms over the side of the table.

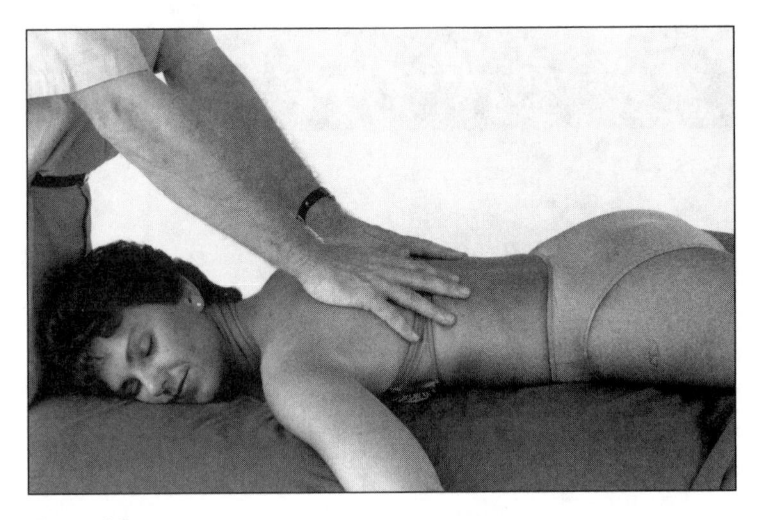

Figure 8.3

The Work: Breath Release Three

Client Position: Prone, with support under the chest

1. Place hands on the scapula and ribcage.

2. Follow the client's breath, compressing on the exhalation.

3. Sense which motion is most restricted; anteriorly or inferiorly.

4. Place emphasis on the restriction.

Functional Breath Release Four

The fourth technique begins with the client in side lying position. Your left hand cradles in the client's axilla, and your top hand cradles over the deltoid, shown in Figure 8.4. Follow the breathing just as you have done in the previous technique, and this time, on the exhalation, check for just medial compression with your left hand. At the same time, compress your left hand toward the spine. Your top hand is compressing the shoulder girdle inferiorly as well as distracting the shoulder girdle laterally. While you are compressing with one hand and distracting with the other, you are actually trying to line up the tumblers in a lock, so to speak, and as you are compressing, you are searching for the angle of release. So the work becomes interesting as you only have the time it takes for the client to exhale. Then let the client inhale unrestricted and continue to search for the vector of release on the second and third exhalation. There is an end feel that is very distinguishable. It often has the sense of something giving an extra quarter of an inch or so as the client gets closer to the end point of the exhalation. Sometimes you can also cue the client at the end point of exhalation: Can you let just a little more air out? Remember not to hold the exhale for more than a couple of seconds, and it is not unusual at all for clients to be waiting for a verbal cue to tell them to inhale, so be mindful of this. You really have to keep track of the client's respiration for her because you are working with it directly. Always be aware of where she is at in her cycle of breath, and to remember that she may be waiting for a reminder from you to breathe. For someone just learning these techniques, that is without a doubt the simplest one and can be the most effective for most of the clients.

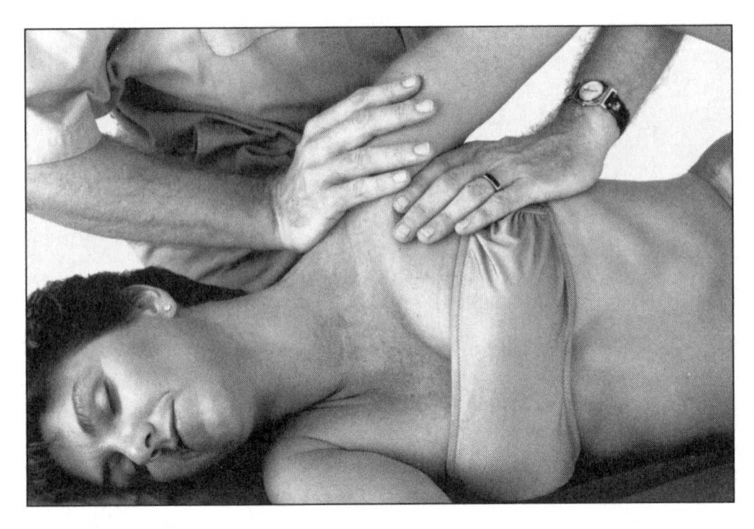

Figure 8.4

The Work: Breath Release Four

Client Position: Side lying, with knees flexed 45°

1. Left hand cradles in client's axilla and right hand cradles over the deltoid.

2. On the client's exhalation, check to see that the client's ribcage is moving down toward the table, and her shoulder is gliding laterally and inferiorly toward her pelvis.

3. Left hand is compressing toward the table as the right hand distracts the shoulder laterally and glides inferiorly.

4. Verbal cues for breath are necessary.

Lung Fissure

The lungs have three fissures in them that separate the various lobes. On the right side there is a horizontal fissure that runs approximately from the mid-coronal plane of the fourth rib all the way to the sternum following a line approximately under the fourth rib. There is also an oblique fissure on both the right and left lungs, and it too runs approximately, starting at the coronal plane and going obliquely from the fourth to the eighth rib. In Figure 8.5the therapist's hand is positioned along the oblique fissure of the right lung. The technique is done by placing your hand along the approximate line of the fissure and applying a compressional force mostly through the edge of your hand along the forefinger and thumb.

Begin the technique by following the client's inhale and apply the compression on her exhale. At the end of the exhale, maintain most of your compressional force while she continues to inhale. After two or three cycles of respiration, you will feel some give in the rib cage as your hand slips more medially toward the spine and inferiorly toward the pelvis. Once you begin to feel this, you know you have got the release. The amount of pressure that you are using is approximately 5 to 10 pounds. It is firm and deep. It is highly recommended to get out your anatomy books and look at the positions of the lung fissures before beginning this technique. You can also see in Figure 8.5 that the therapist has the client turn her head to the opposite side that he is working. This will help stretch the entire pleura. You will find this technique especially valuable for any clients who have orthopedic injuries around the trunk or respiratory problems in general, and anyone who has had a history of broken or fractured ribs.

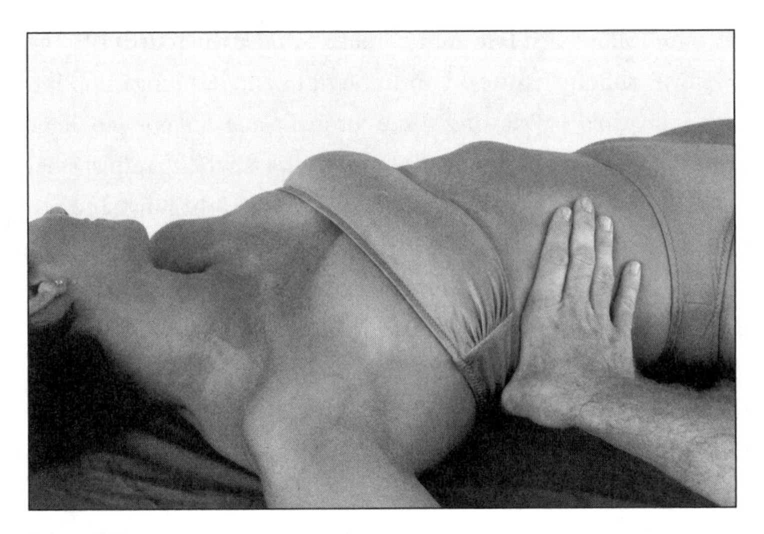

Figure 8.5

The Work: Lung Fissure

Client Position: Supine

First hand position is on the oblique fissure of the right lung.

Apply compressional force with 5 to 10 pounds of pressure through the edge of the hand along the four fingers and thumb.

Follow the client's inhale and apply compressional force on the exhale.

At the end of the exhale, maintain most of the compressional force while she continues to inhale.

Wait for a softening and then repeat to the horizontal fissure on the right side.

Then repeat to the oblique fissure on the left side.

Costovertebral and Costotransverse Joints

Figures 8.6 and 8.7 show a very gentle, easy, and even pleasurable stretch that you can do with clients. It is good to use this technique any time you do work around the ribs on the back. With the client sitting up with her feet hanging off the table, have her grasp her fingertips together and place them in the back of her neck. Her elbows should be as close together as possible. With your left arm, hook her elbows from underneath and ask the client to give you her bodyweight on top of your arm. Your back hand is on the spine at mid-back as shown in Figure 8.6. Once you have a sense that she has given you her weight, begin to slowly backward bend the client and take her into extension. This is done slowly with your right hand applying several pounds of anterior compression on the vertebrae. Apply the technique while she is exhaling. Finish the technique by bringing her back up to center and replacing your hand higher or lower on her spine. You could also start at the top and work down or vice versa. However, one pivot point seems to be where the dorsal vertebrae and thoracic vertebrae meet the lumbarvertebrae. Besides placing pressure on the spine, Figure 8.7 also shows the therapist placing pressure on the posterior angle of the ribs. This is a great stretch, and it is not unusual to hear some snap, crackle, or pop, so do not be frightened if you hear noise. This is a very nonspecific mobilization that helps integrate soft tissue work into the bony skeleton. Alternately, you can do an unwinding or spiral type motion slowly as long as the client feels comfortable giving you her weight on your opposite hand that is supporting her elbows. By this you can not only backward bend the client, but side-bend her to one side and the other. Then begin to circumduct her whole trunk first to the right and then to the left. In this way, you can feel where various snags and restrictions are in the fascial planes, and it is useful information for future reference.

Unwinding always has three vectors that you are searching for. In this position, you are checking flexion-extension, side-bending,

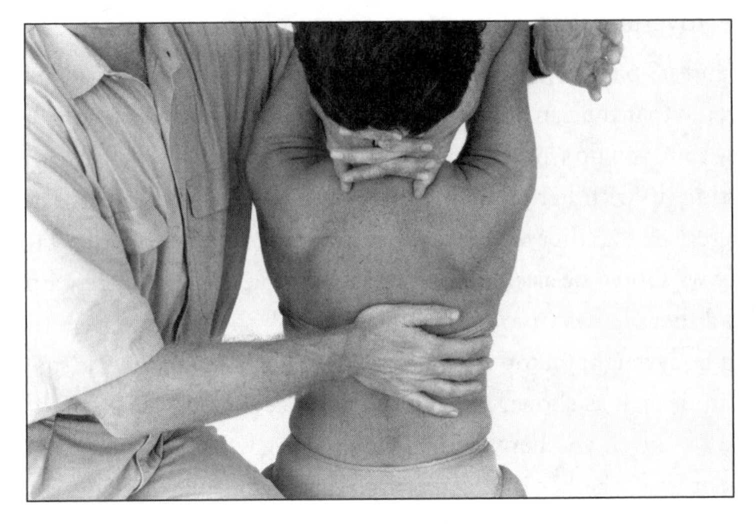

Figure 8.6

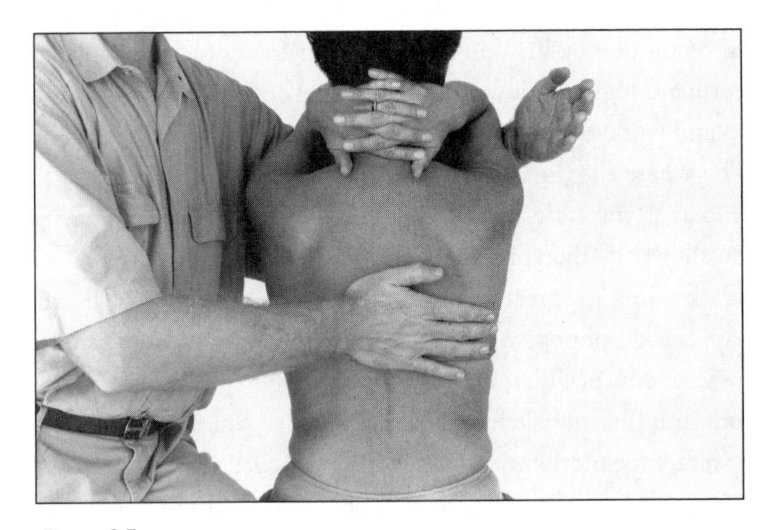

Figure 8.7

and rotation. There are two styles of unwinding. The first is to follow the path of least resistance in each of those three vectors. You listen for barriers and stopping points, wait, hold, and follow each release along its least resistant path. The second style of unwinding is to stack up those three vectors against the restriction barrier. Let us say that you test the spine for flexion/extension, and it feels more restricted going into extension. You hold it in extension and test for side-bending, and it is tighter on the right so you hold it to the right and then you twist the spine clockwise and counterclockwise. If it is stuck going clockwise, you hold the position. Thus, you have stacked the three restriction barriers and then you wait for a release. You can advance to the next barrier and continue the unwinding. Unwinding has diminishing returns after several minutes. This is because the receptors in the fascia of the autonomic nervous system can become overstimulated.

The Work: Costovertebral and Costotransverse Joints

Client Position: Sitting upright at the edge of the table

1. Client grasps fingertips together and places them at the back of her neck with her elbows as close together as possible.

2. Place left arm under client's elbows, asking the client to give her body weight.

3. Right hand is placed mid-back over the spine.

4. Remind the client to gently give her body weight to you.

5. Slowly backbend the client into extension on the exhale.

6. As the client exhales, right hand applies several pounds of anterior compression into the vertebra.

7. Bring the client back to neutral.

8. Place right hand higher or lower on the spine and repeat the sequence.

9. In addition, pressure can be applied to the posterior angle of the ribs.

10. If the client feels comfortable, take her into lateral flexion and rotation.

11. Three Vectors—Flexion/extension, side-bending, rotation

12. The first is to find the path of least resistance, hold and then relax.

    a. The second is to stack up the three vectors against the restriction, and wait for releases.

Costochondral and Costosternal Joint Spaces

You can see in Figure 8.8 that the therapist has overlapped his thumbs and placed them over the costosternal joint space. That is the joint space where the rib meets the sternum. The idea in this technique is to apply a slight 5-pound compression posteriorly into that joint space while the client is exhaling. Maintain your pressure on the ribs as the client inhales. Just let up your pressure a little bit and do this for three cycles of respiration, and you will find the rib house begin to loosen up. It may be a bit excessive to repeat this process over each and every joint space, whether it is the costosternal or costochondral joint that is just an inch lateral to the sternum on the rib. Instead, you may wish to palpate each of these joint spaces with less pressure and choose those ribs that are the most fixated. A rib that is fixated feels very dense and hard. When compressing a rib or a joint space of a rib, there should definitely be some give to it, and if not, you can be rest assured that the rib is fixated. You will like this technique because it also accesses the client's respiration. In reality, the client is doing the work; you are just assisting the process by using her respiratory mechanism. In addition, you can jiggle or

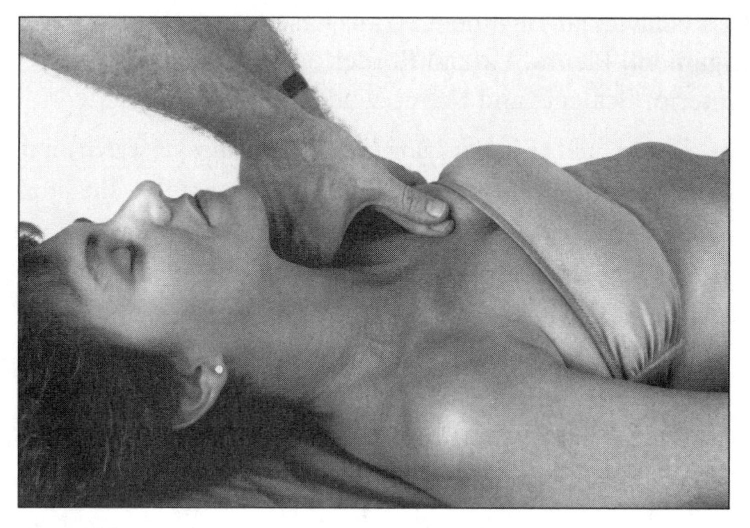

Figure 8.8

bounce the rib occasionally during your compression. This helps to vibrate the joint space and aid in its release. Have the client focus her inhale on the point of contact, and when she reaches the peak of her inhale, lighten up your pressure briefly before the next compression.

The Work: Costochondral and Costosternal Joint Spaces

Client Position: Supine

1. Place thumbs over costosternal joint space.

2. Apply slight 5-pound compression posteriorly while the client is exhaling.

3. Maintain pressure while the client inhales; lighten pressure to accommodate the breath.

4. Repeat for three cycles of respiration to feel a softening.

5. Repeat to ribs that are fixated until a softening is felt.

Costoclavicular Ligament, Transverse Clavicular Ligament, Pleura, Lateral Border of Trapezius, Anterior Scalene, and Sternocleidomastoid

The client should be in side lying position. Begin your search on the superior border of the clavicle as shown in Figure 8.9. The proximal third of clavicle accesses the anterior scalene, costoclavicular ligament, and the transverse clavicular ligament. The middle third accesses the clavipectoral fascia and dome of the pleura (cupula of pleura and suprapleural membrane—scalene fascia/Simpson's fascia). To get directly onto the pleura, go to the middle of the clavicle so that the fingertips are pointing directly into the lungs. Wait and maintain pressure until pleura softens. Continue to search the distal end of the clavicle for fibers of the trapezius and trapezoid ligament. It is important to remember that you must move the clavicle with your opposite (supporting) hand superiorly to gain deeper access to the above-mentioned structures. You must go slowly, waiting, holding, and moving in unison with the client's breath. You can also friction to release the pleural dome.

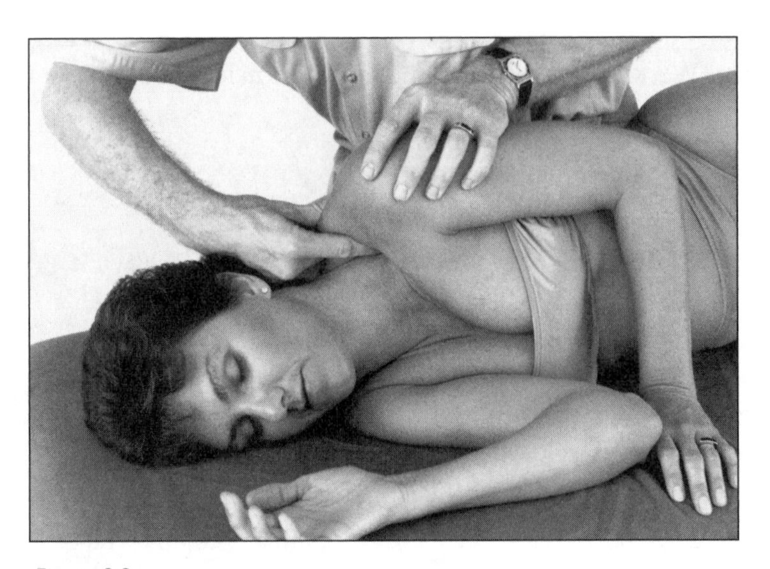

Figure 8.9

The Work: Costoclavicular Ligament, Transverse Clavicular Ligament, Pleura, Lateral Border of Trapezius, Anterior Scalene, and Sternocleidomastoid

Client Position: Side lying, with knees flexed 45°

1. Begin on the superior border of the proximal third of the clavicle.

2. Move medially to access all tissues, being mindful of the brachial plexus that lies in between anterior and middle scalene.

3. Wait and maintain pressure until all tissues soften while moving the clavicle superiorly with the supporting hand.

4. Move slowly and in unison with the client's breath.

5. Friction to release the plural dome.

Serratus Posterior Superior and Inferior and the Levatores Costarum Muscles

Figure 8.10 demonstrates the beginning of a long sequence of work on the levatores costarum and serratus posterior inferior muscles. The client is side-lying with her head supported and her knees flexed to a 45° angle. It is also recommended to place a pillow or towel between the client's knees to help support her. The entry point for this technique, shown in Figure 8.10, is going to be in an area on top of the posterior inferior serratus muscle. This muscle attaches to ribs 9–12, thereby affecting the floating ribs, specifically the twelfth rib. There are a wide variety of structures that attach to the twelfth rib, namely the quadratus lumborum, the peritoneum, the latissimus dorsi, the erectors, the posterior inferior serratus, the diaphragm, the two layers of pleura, the internal and

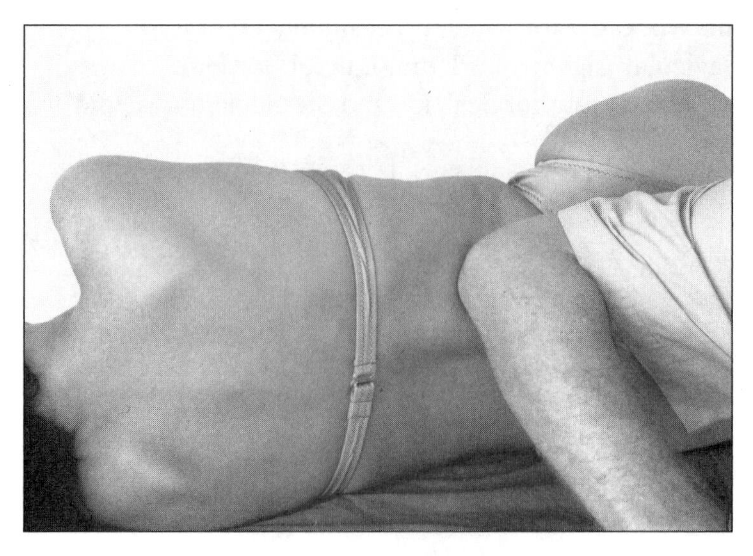

Figure 8.10

external intercostals, as well as the deep ligamentus structures of the erector group. There is a whole lot going on in this area, and in many cases, the twelfth rib, because of low back problems, has been pulled down by the quadratus lumborum much closer toward the crest of the ilium and as such is contributing to the low back problem. Serratus posterior inferior assists in lifting the ribs during inhalation. There is also some speculation that the posterior serratus muscle acts as a type of retinaculum for the erector spinae muscles. This technique is somewhat vigorous and requires that you pay full attention to the client's breathing and also maintain verbal contact with her throughout.

The position is kneeling on the floor using your right elbow on the edge of the erectors at the bottom of the ribs. You can find what position works for you. You will have already palpated with your hand where the bottom of the ribs are as well as the approximate location of the floating ribs, especially the twelfth rib. Place your elbow in the area of the floating ribs and press directly anteriorly with 10 to 15 pounds of pressure. This is a particularly sensitive area

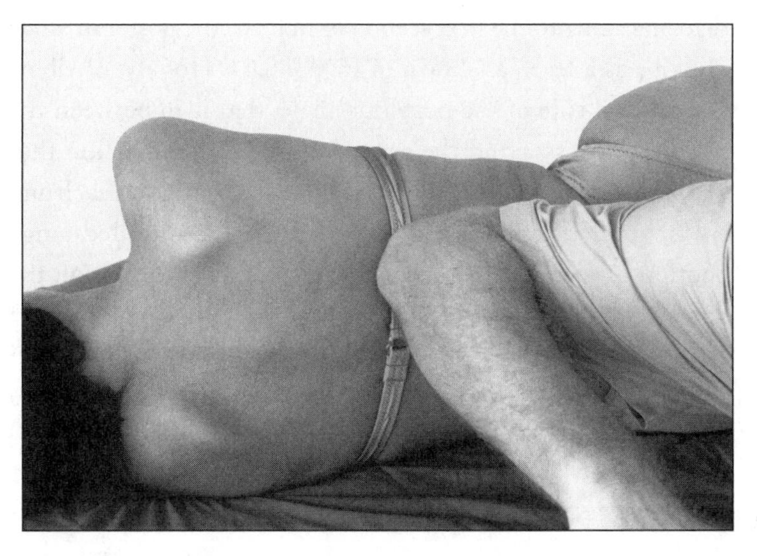

Figure 8.11

of the body, and your movements need to be done very slowly and very evenly. The attempt is to friction the short ligaments and deep muscle fibers over the floating ribs. When you do this, it should be done on an inhalation. You can also ask the client to tuck her tailbone forward and that will bring her spine back toward you, and give you a broader surface to work on. Once you have frictioned the area two or three times, stop and move on to the next section of ribs higher up. However, before you move on, make sure that the client takes a deep breath into the area that you just worked. Have the client take a slow full breath into the area after each time you make a pass in the tissue. Each pass into the tissue should only be 15–30 seconds in length, given the potential intensity of the technique. There is a hallmark that a floating rib has freedom: during inhalation you will see in the side lying position, if you step away from the client, that the hip will move inferiorly and the trunk will move superiorly, causing the waistline of the client to gap open. Check this motion before you even begin to work, so that you have some motion to reference when you finish the technique.

Moving along to the next section of ribs, use the posterior angle of the ribs as a lever, as shown in Figure 8.11. Hook your elbow on the medial side of the posterior angle, that is in between the transverse processes and the posterior angle. Then friction that posterior angle several times. You do not need to friction each and every rib, but only those ribs that you feel have a limited range of motion. Another variation of this technique is to friction the erectors in the lamina groove at those areas of the spine that are particularly tight or thickened with very dense tissue. It should also be remembered that the posterior layer of the lumbar fascia extends from the sacrum all the way up to the cervicals. In this way, you are working not only ribs and erectors, but also the entire paraspinal fascial system.

As the therapist moves on to the upper ribs, in Figure 8.12, you will see that the client has her arm extended to the front, toward the wall, including her shoulder with the movement. Very often when you ask the client to reach with her arm, she won't move her shoulder. The best way to facilitate the proper movement is to cue her to lengthen her entire arm, coaching her to stretch first through her fingertips, her elbow, and up her shoulder while reaching to the wall and even down to the floor. This will abduct the scapula, exposing the posterior angle of the ribs on the upper trunk. Serratus posterior superior lives here under the rhomboids and attaches to the dorsal midline fascia. To search for adhesions in this muscle, have the client abduct the scapula even further by reaching toward the wall and then down to the floor. According to the Travell and Simons manuals, a hidden trigger point can be found here that produces extremely deep upper back pain (Travell & Simons, 1998). An alternative to this, if the client can handle it, is to have her reach with her forehead toward her knees and that will extend the tissue of the neck and upper dorsals and further contribute to any release that goes on in the upper extremities. Give yourself at least 15 to 20 minutes on each side of the back to do this work.

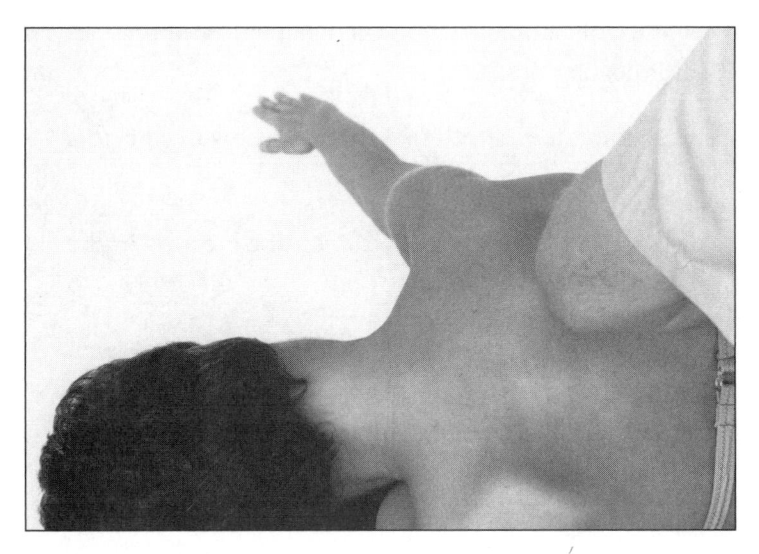

Figure 8.12

Note, you need to give the client lots of break time by letting her breathe or go through two or three cycles of respiration every 3 to 4 minutes. Breaks will allow time for her nervous system to settle down from the input. It is important to keep in mind that directly on the anterior surface of the ribs are the sympathetic nervous system ganglia.

The Work: Serratus Posterior Superior and Inferior and Levatores Costarum

Client Position: Side lying, with knees flexed 45°

1. Place right elbow on the edge of erectors at the bottom of the ribs facing the client's head.

2. Direction of force is anterior using 10 to 15 pounds of pressure.

3. Keep pressure even and enter slowly.

4. On inhalation, friction the ligaments and muscles over floating ribs.

5. Ask for deep breath into the area just worked before moving on superiorly.

6. Another variation is to friction the erectors in the lamina groove.

7. Moving onto the upper ribs, ask the client to reach toward the wall and down to the floor to abduct the scapula and continue searching for active adhesions.

8. Movements to ask for:

- Tuck tailbone forward
- Chin to chest
- Arm to wall
- Arm down to floor
- Breath

Serratus Anterior and the Clavipectoral Fascia

This technique is a convenient way to work the serratus anterior. It also is a comprehensive release for the clavipectoral fascia. With the client in side lying, have her bend her arm and point her elbow to the ceiling at a perpendicular angle to the table. Gently rest the point of your elbow in the axilla as you can see in Figure 8.13, most of the lower part of the therapist's forearm is on top of the coronal plane of the client. The therapist is directly over and has under his elbow almost all of the serratus anterior. Begin to apply a slow, even compression into the ribs medially toward the spine. At the same time, have the client lift the point of her elbow up to the ceiling. Repeat this process two or three times while maintaining medial compression toward the table. Add a second vector gliding several inches at a time toward the pelvis while the client takes her elbow to the ceiling and then slowly

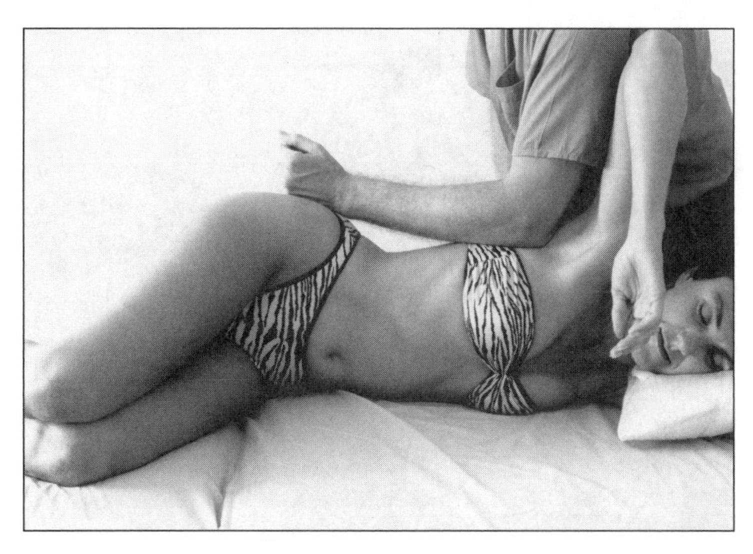

Figure 8.13

over her head. You can also friction when you find a particularly stuck area. Always work with the client's respiration and have her use her breath as an ally in this particular work. Stay connected to the serratus for 30–45 seconds at a time. You can cross fiber every now and then. The important thing to remember is to have the client push her breath into where you are working to mobilize the ribs.

The Work: Serratus Anterior and the Clavipectoral Fascia

Client Position: Side lying, with knees flexed 45°

1. The client's elbow points to the celling at a 90°angle.

2. Facing client's feet, rest elbow in the client's axilla.

3. Apply a slow even compression to the ribs.

4. While the client's elbow lifts to the ceiling, wait for a softening, asking for an occasional breath.

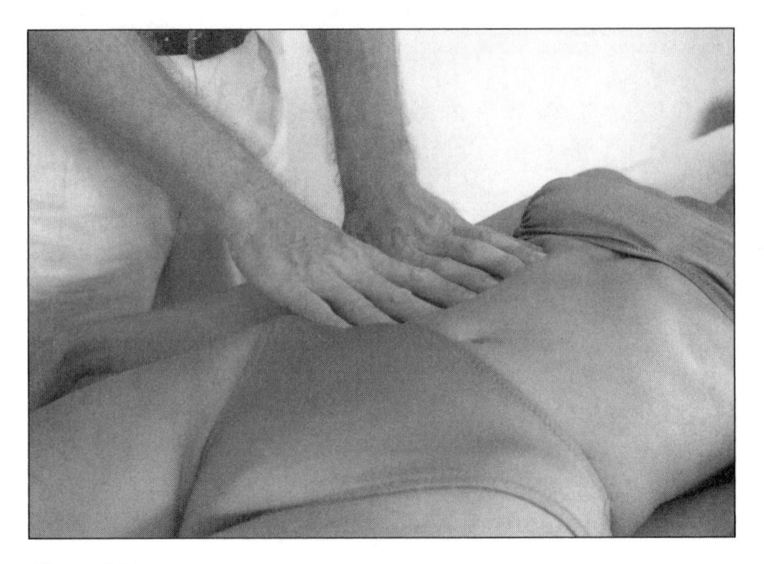

Figure 8.14

5. Repeat two to three times.

6. A second vector can be added with a gliding to the pelvis as the client's elbow reaches over the head.

7. Ask the client for respiration.

8. Friction when necessary.

9. Repeat two to three times.

Ventral Fascia over the Rectus Abdominus and the Costal Arch

The fascia over the rectus, which is called the ventral fascia of the body, has a tendency to migrate laterally when it loses its integrity. Fascia of the body loses its integrity in any number of different ways. It can be caused by poor nutrition, overexercise, underexercise, postsurgical adhesion, neurological trauma, and especially orthopedic trauma. This technique creates organization in the fascia over and around the rectus abdominus. As shown in Figure 8.14, place your fingertips several inches lateral of the umbilicus in an area lateral to the rectus abdominus. Allow your fingers to sink into the abdomen so that you can imagine that you are going to lift the rectus abdominus muscle up from underneath. Then start very slowly, moving the tissue toward the midline, toward the umbilicus of the body. When you arrive at the midline, let go and start over again. This procedure can be repeated several times in one place before moving below or above. This is also a good stretch for the peritoneum. Work one side at a time, spending anywhere from 5 to 10 minutes on each side doing this kind of work over the rectus.

In Figure 8.15, the therapist is working bilaterally over the costal arch of the client. However, you could also do this one side at a time. Remember that the rectus abdominus attaches to the fifth rib, and the fifth rib is almost at midsternum. The therapist's fingers are spread wide and start lateral on the edge of the rib cage. The therapist works at an angle, bringing the tissue toward the sternum. Any technique done on or around the rib cage is going to be twofold in practice. This means that first and foremost, you need to be making contact with the ribs and pressing into the ribs, mobilizing the ribs in order to free respiration. Second is the movement of the tissue that you are working on, and in this case, it is the fascia of the rectus abdominus. This technique then involves finding the first vector, going into the ribs, pressing into the lungs and pleura incrementally with several pounds of pressure, and then moving into the second vector and taking the tissue toward the midline. The movement that the therapist solicits in the client is to have her lift her head occasionally, activating the rectus abdominus. You can also ask the client to flex her knee, or occasionally you could ask her to lift her whole leg up very slightly off the table and then relax it. One of the things consistently seen while doing this technique is that the shape of the rectus abdominus will change and it will lengthen.

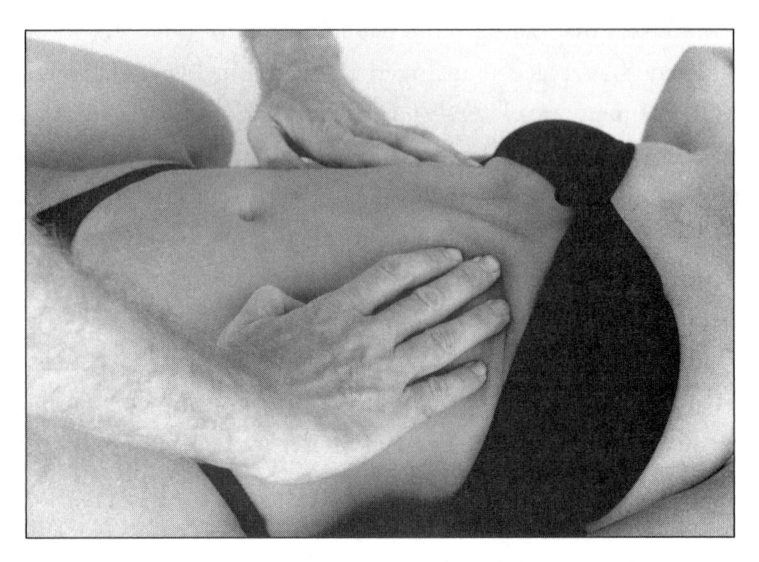

Figure 8.15

Also, after several minutes of this work over the costal arch, you will begin to see the trunk lift and the diaphragm expand. The other thing that is important to remember when working around the rib cage is to ask the client to take a breath occasionally, not only into your hands at the point of contact while you are working, but also when you take a break every minute or so. This will be especially true as you work down into the lower abdomen and have the client breathe down into the lower abdomen, which very few people do. See more about asking for breath in Tips on Asking for Movement.

The Work: Ventral Fascia over the Rectus Abdominus

Client Position: Supine

1 Place fingers several inches lateral to the umbilicus.

2. Let fingers sink into the belly as if trying to lift the rectus abdominus from underneath.

3. Move tissues toward the midline.

4. Upon arriving at the midline, release, and start over again.

The Work: Ventral Fascia over the Costal Arch

Client Position: Supine

1. Place fingers bilaterally onto the costal arch or work one side at a time.

2. Vector into the ribs and mobilize the ribs.

3. Once a softening is felt, take the tissues toward the midline or against its restriction barrier while asking for movement.

4. Movements to ask for are:

- Lift head
- Flex knee
- Lift whole leg off the table slightly
- Breath, occasionally

Rectus Abdominus over the Pubic Symphysis

This technique starts off searching for trigger points on the pubic symphysis. Normally when you look for a trigger point, you are looking for an area of tenderness as reported by the client, as well as an area of restriction or tightness. Figure 8.16 shows a skeletal view of the pubic symphysis. Before beginning your search, ask the client to find her own pubic symphysis bone. You might have to do some verbal coaching. Once she has made contact with the pubic symphysis, place your fingers over hers as shown in Figure 8.17. Now you have the option to work over her hand, or she can remove her hand and you will be right on the bone. This eliminates the need to search for the client's pubic symphysis as this is a vulnerable area for most clients.

Start by placing both of your thumbs or finger pads down on the midline of the symphysis and press posteriorly with a pound or two of pressure. Always apply pressure very slowly and incrementally, working up to a pound or two of pressure if necessary. It is important to be in verbal contact with the client at this point, asking each time you press into her symphysis if that area is tender. If it is not tender, move to the left or right of the symphysis a quarter of an inch at a time, searching for trigger points. You need only go at most an inch and a half on either side of the midline. Take no more than 3 to 5 minutes looking for these trigger points. Once you find the trigger point, hold the trigger point for 30 to 45 seconds until you feel it soften, or until the client reports that she feels no more pain. These trigger points for the rectus abdominus can also be reflexing into the floor of the pelvis, and especially the bladder, which is directly underneath the pubic bone. As an alternative, you can friction the rectus abdominus over the pubic bone, and again do this slowly on either side. The movement you can ask for while working in this delicate area is to have the client lift her head up or to have her lift her leg or flex her knees alternately, first her left and then her right.

All of this work on the rectus abdominus, as well as the quadriceps, is important to do before even attempting to palpate the psoas. The quadriceps often overpower the lower part of the psoas and its attachment on the lesser trochanter of the femur. The same is true for the rectus abdominus, because in this culture there is an inappropriate attempt to overstrengthen and overfortify the muscles of the rectus abdominus in order to support the lower back. There is no sense trying to palpate the psoas through the abdomen if the rectus abdominus is too tight. You may eventually spend 30 to 45 minutes doing this type of work over the rectus abdominus and each one of the quadriceps before you even make an attempt to palpate the psoas. You may need to repeat this work over the rectus and the quads over a period of several treatments before attempting to get into the psoas, so do not be disheartened by this type of delay. Use indirect techniques for the psoas if you cannot work through the rectus abdominus.

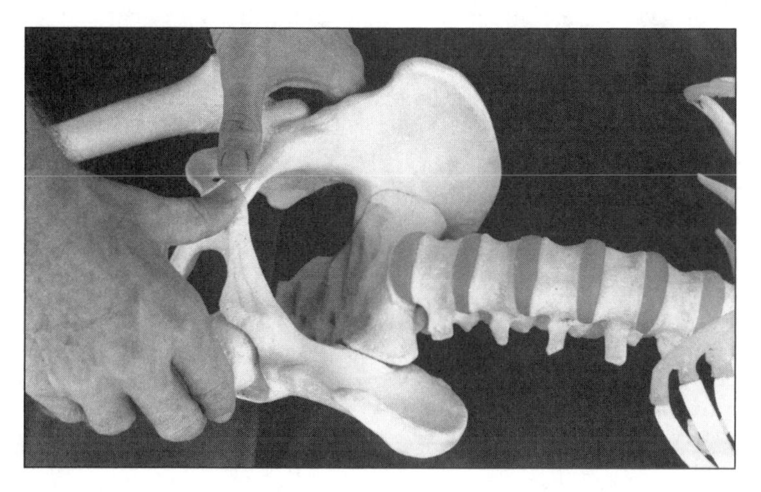

Figure 8.16

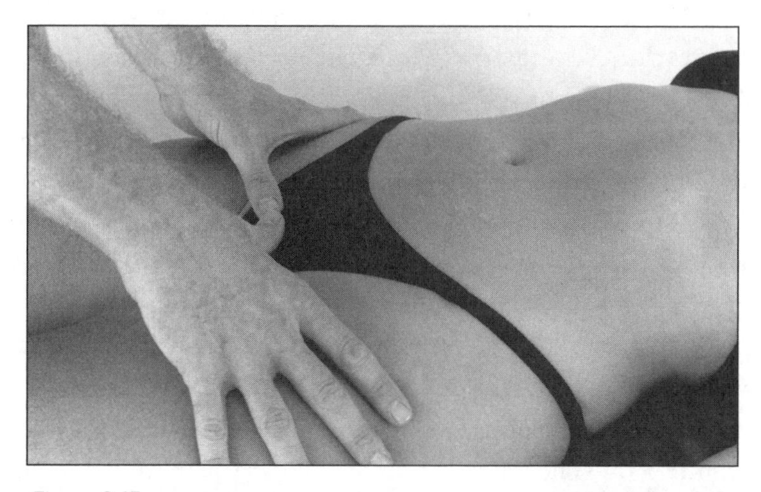

Figure 8.17

The Work: Rectus Abdominus over the Pubic Symphysis

Client Position: Supine

1. Ask the client to find her own pubic symphysis.

2. Place thumbs down on the midline of the pubic symphysis and press in with a pound or two of pressure.

3. Apply pressure slowly.

4. Move medially and laterally along the ridge searching for trigger points, holding 30 to 45 seconds until a softening. Friction if necessary.

5. Stay in verbal contact.

6. Movements to ask for are:

    - Lift head
    - Lift leg alternately
    - Flex knee alternately

Iliopsoas Muscle

This technique is very direct work on the iliopsoas. It is important that the client be seated on a bench with her feet flat on the ground. While her feet are flat on the ground, her hips need to be on the same plane with her knees, or slightly higher. In other words, if her knees are above her hip, elevate her pelvis. The feet need to be spread hip-width apart, and she needs to be seated straight up with her arms relaxed down at her sides. Place your fingers lateral and inferior to the umbilicus and into the abdomen. Notice in Figure 8.18 that the angle of the therapist's hands is toward the spine as well as straight back into the abdomen. You are always looking for at least two vectors of release, and therefore your hands always go into the body. When the tight tissue is found, you move at another

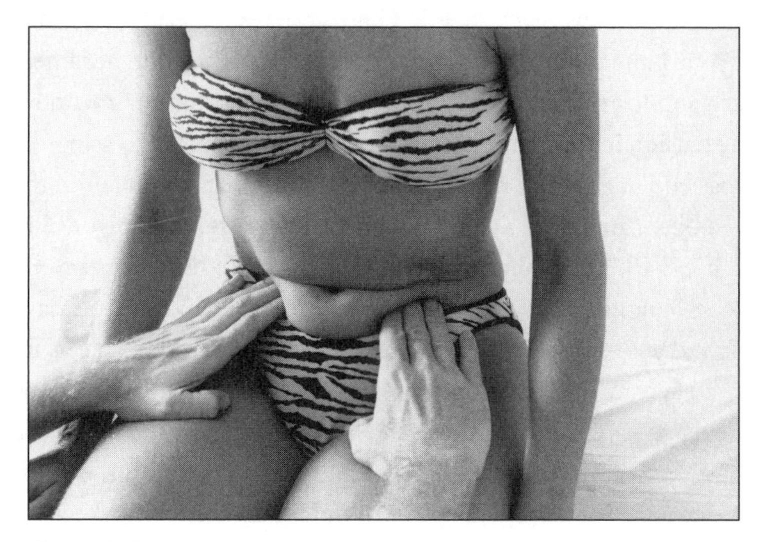

Figure 8.18

angle to get proper leverage. Enter the abdomen just an inch or two, without much pressure, and then ask the client to slowly bend forward several inches and then have her stop. Allow your fingers to sink into the abdomen a little bit more, and then have the client bend over several inches until her head is hanging about half way to her knees. Then have her stop. Make sure that her arms are hanging down at the sides of her knees and not holding on to anything. At this point, allow your pressure to move fully back toward the posterior abdominal wall and make contact with the psoas. If you're not sure you're making contact with the psoas, have the client lift one foot off the ground. It can be either her right or her left. You will feel the psoas pop right into your fingers. Repeat this with the opposite leg. Then repeat the whole procedure several times on either side. Use your fingertips to friction the psoas and hold on to the psoas. On your last attempt at the psoas, have the client sit back up straight and take a deep breath while you hold on to the psoas. Disengage slowly.

Figure 8.19 shows an alternative client position for this work. With the client in supine position, have her bring her knees up and spread her feet widely so that her knees can rest together. Place one of your hands over both of her knees and gently jiggle her knees back and forth so that her legs can rest and relax together without any tension in the legs. This will be very beneficial to accessing the psoas and to getting a better release if there is no tension left in the legs. Next, approach the psoas the same way the therapist did in Figure 8.18, with your fingers just lateral to the umbilicus several inches, angling down and in toward the spine. When you have allowed your fingers to sink posteriorly or down to the table as far as you can go, have the client lift her foot off the table on the same side as you are working. Once she lifts her foot up, the psoas will pop right into your fingers. Then maintain contact with the psoas on one side and have her slowly straighten her leg while keeping her heel several inches off the table. You can also have the client press through her heel, which helps lengthen the line from the psoas down to the foot. Repeat this on the opposite side and then make an evaluation of which psoas is larger, which psoas is tighter, and where the relative position of each psoas is. Upon evaluation of which side is tighter, repeat this several times. Each time you work in the abdomen, remove your hands and ask the client to take a breath into where you just worked.

> Breathing is an essential part of the psoas technique. The respiratory diaphragm shares an attachment with the psoas.

The Work: Iliopsoas

Client Position: Seated, with feet flat on the ground and hips level with knees or slightly higher

1. Kneel directly in front of the client.
2. Place fingers lateral to the umbilicus into the belly.

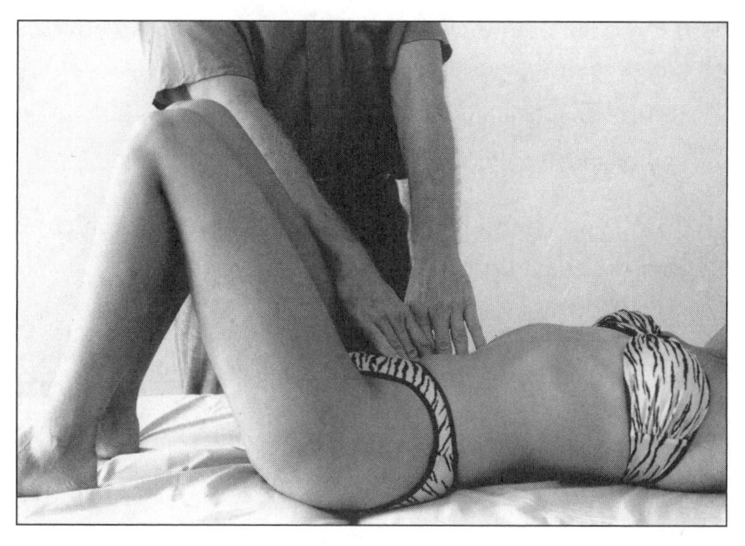

Figure 8.19

3. Enter into the belly gently and ask the client to bend forward slightly.

4. Enter the tissues more deeply and have the client bend even more until her head is hanging slightly and everything including her arms is relaxed.

5. Move more posteriorly and make contact with the psoas muscle.

6. If unsure contact with the muscle has been made, have the client lift one foot off the ground. The psoas will jump right into fingers.

7. Repeat this process asking her to lift the opposite leg.

8. Friction psoas when necessary and repeat this process a couple of times.

9. On the last attempt, have the client sit back up straight and take a deep breath while holding on to psoas.

Client Position: Supine with knees bent, feet spread apart with knees resting together gently

1. Place gentle fingers just lateral to the umbilicus several inches and angle down toward the spine.

2. When fingers are woven as posteriorly as possible, have the client lift her foot off of the table.

3. Hold on to the psoas and ask the client to straighten her leg keeping her heel several inches off the table. Once there, ask her to press through her heel.

4. Assess which side is tighter and repeat several times.

5. Ask for breath each time hand contact is released.

Quadratus Lumborum

The quadratus lumborum is perhaps the most important muscle in the low back. It attaches along the transverse processes of the lumbar vertebrae and also to the crest of the ilium and the twelfth rib. When the quadratus gets short or loses its tone because of problems with the spine and low back, it will pull the twelfth rib down out of its position and move it toward the crest of the ilium, and sometimes underneath the crest toward the iliacus muscle. Ida Rolf felt that the most frequently distorted structure in the human body and one of the most important structures in the human body was the twelfth rib. This little rib has many different structures attaching to it, including the diaphragm, the pleura, the lattisimus dorsi, the erectors, the posterior inferior serratus, the quadratus, and the rotatores to name a few. It is very important if you are working with low back syndrome to place a portion of your emphasis on lifting the twelfth rib.

Figure 8.20 shows the therapist with his elbow over the floating rib. Use a broad contact and move the tissue from lateral to medial

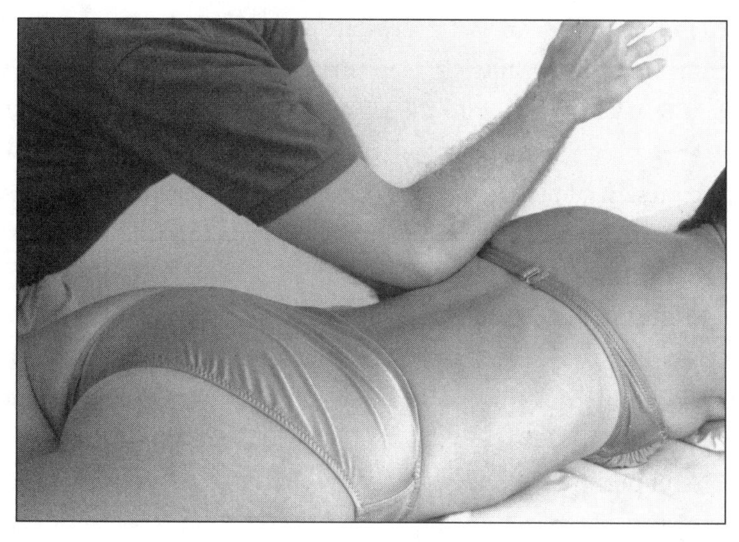

Figure 8.20

at a slight diagonal with the vector toward the opposite shoulder. This goes against the grain of the two rules of thumb presented on organizing the paraspinal fascia; however, this is one of the few exceptions to the rule. You can understand how important it is to lift that floating rib, and it is hoped that you spend time palpating the floating rib on all low back clients. You will be astounded at where they are located and at how much tissue they are buried under. You can move the tissue from lateral to medial at that diagonal line toward the opposite shoulder, and repeat this two or three times. Then what you may like to do is prop the client up on her elbows, as you can see in Figure 8.21. Start just slightly above the floating rib and place the point of your elbow right in the middle of each erector and slowly apply compression into the muscle and then glide down toward the sacrum several inches at a time. Most of your low back clients are kyphotic and over a period of time have lost their curvature. This is a terrific position to reintroduce normal curvature into the lumbars, and also to lengthen the erectors, quadratus lumborum, and floating ribs. You can repeat this process two to three times on each side, starting with a light pressure and gradually building up to a deep pressure. Again, always ask the client to take a breath into the area you just worked on, especially the area of the floating ribs, since you are trying to mobilize those structures. In addition, while the client is propped up on her elbows, you can have her lift her tailbone slightly, and this will also assist in establishing appropriate curvature.

Figure 8.21 also shows the therapist working with his elbow in the middle layer or septum between the erectors and the quadratus lumborum. This is a repeat of the previous work just done in prone position, except now he is placing the client in a more stressful position and using an elbow that has considerably more force available to it. Remember that any pain that becomes exacerbated from the technique or is elicited from the technique is a contraindication to doing this particular release or any techniques for that matter.

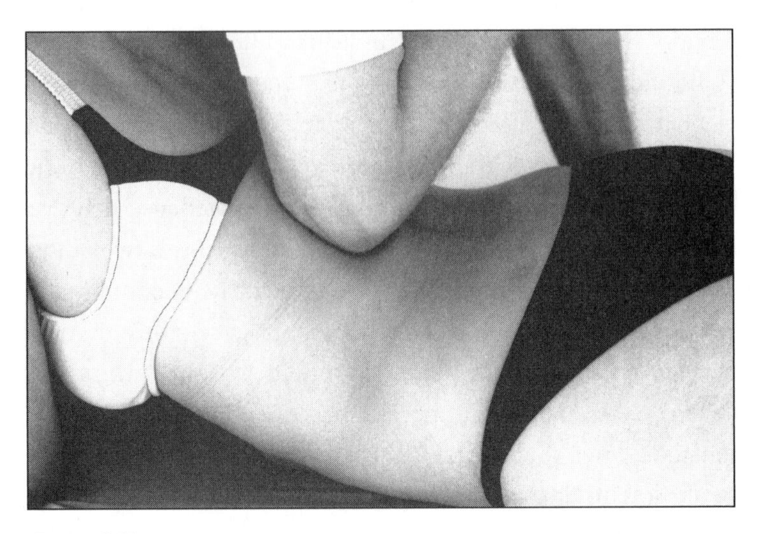

Figure 8.21

If the client has too much lordosis, having the client up on her elbows is contraindicated. Instead, to perform this same release without encouraging more lordosis, put her in a child's pose position; the body facing the table in fetal position. Draping would require extra attention and you may need a step stool to perform the release.

The Work: Quadratus Lumborum

Client Position: Prone

1. Make broad contact over the twelfth rib and move the tissue from lateral to medial at a slight diagonal vector toward the opposite shoulder, repeating two to three times.

2. Prop the client up on her elbows and place the elbow right in the middle of the erectors just slightly above the floating rib.

3. Apply compression into the muscle and glide inferiorly toward the sacrum.

4. Repeat two or three times on each side.

5. Movements to ask for are:

   - Pelvic tilts
   - Breath into the area
   - Lengthen the femur bone

6. Being mindful of the use of force, the septum in between the erectors and the QL can be worked with the client in extension.

7. The client can move up to elbows or in to the child's pose position upon evaluation.

Surface Anatomy of the Sacrum

This describes some of the topographical features and anatomical details of the sacrum. A basic view of the positioning of the sacrum is modeled in Figure 8.22.The sacrum has at least seven biomechanical axes of motion and a variety of soft tissue structures that attach to it from above and below. It also is the lower pole of the parasympathetic nervous system. The sacro-coccygeal plexus, or as some anatomists call it, the splanchnic nerve, come out of the anterior surface of the sacrum to innervate the floor of the pelvis and its organs. The sacrum articulates with the fifth lumbar vertebra from above and with the two ilia on its lateral sides at the sacroiliac joints. In the Figure 8.23 you can see a flat smooth surface on either side of the sacrum, which is the sacroiliac joint. Below the sacroiliac joint, the sacrum begins to narrow as it gets closer to the coccyx, and the narrowing is called the inferior lateral angle of the sacrum, or the ILA. The ligamentous structures are mainly four in number, and there are, of course, others. The superior portion of the sacrum, or the base of the sacrum, which articulates with the fifth lumbar, has the iliolumbar ligaments that go from the transverse processes of the fifth lumbar vertebra to the sacrum and posterior superior iliac spine. The sacroiliac ligament is actually a series of three ligaments, two posterior and one anterior. The two posterior sacroiliac ligaments have horizontal as well as longitudinal fibers. Below the sacroiliac ligament is the bilateral sacrospinous ligament at the ILA, and below the sacrospinous ligaments are the bilateral sacrotuberous ligaments that go down to the tuberosity. There are lateral, posterior, and anterior coccygeal ligaments as well. The most important soft tissue structure that attaches to the sacrum is the piriformis, and it attaches on the anterior surface of the sacrum. Also on the anterior surface of the sacrum are various pelvis diaphragm ligaments that anchor the bladder, the uterus, the cervix, the prostate, and the rectum. This other half, the anterior surface of the sacrum and its many pelvic visceral attachments, is often forgotten.

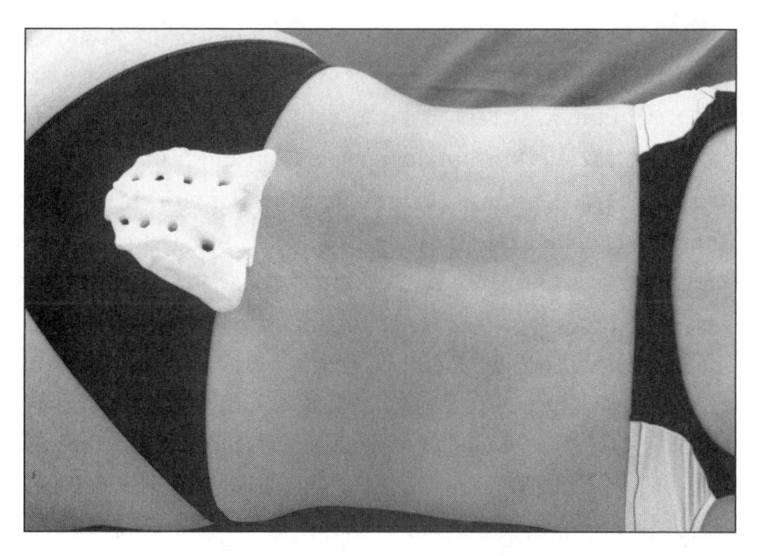

Figure 8.22

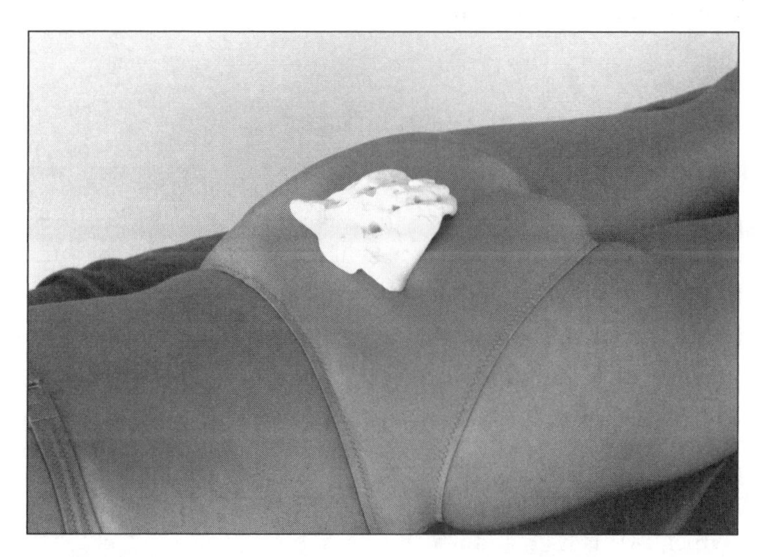

Figure 8.23

Three transverse axes of motion that go through S-1, S-2, and S-3 are considered to be nonphysiologic and appear when the sacrum is out of alignment. The normal transverse axis is through S-2. It is around this axis that the motion of respiration and cranial rhythmic impulse take place. There is a longitudinal axis right down the center of the sacrum that allows rotational movement to occur. There are two oblique axes that go from the right shoulder to the left ischial tuberosity (through the sacrum) and from the left shoulder to the right ischial tuberosity. When one walks, the hamstrings alternately contract and relax. This causes the sacrotuberous ligaments to alternately contract as well. This in turn causes the sacrum to rotate around the oblique axes. Finally, there is an anterior/posterior plane of motion in the sacrum. It can be drawn anteriorly by the pelvic viscera that attaches to it or is pulled posteriorly by the sacral ligaments and biomechanics of the thoracolumbar fascia.

Sacrum: Anterior and Posterior Ligaments

Before working on the sacrum and doing any release work with the sacrum, it is vitally important to determine its biomechanical position. Very often the sacrum will have one side or the other that is dipped lower, and quite often there is a torsion pattern in it as well. You can place your thumbs on each of the sacroiliac joints and alternately compress with several ounces of pressure into each joint space. Figure 8.24 shows the therapist using his thumbs and 8.25 shows the therapist using his whole hand to motion test both the sacroiliac joints as well as the entire sacrum. This gives an idea of which side is high and which side is low as well as a feel for the tissue density over the joint space. You can also determine from this test whether or not the base of the sacrum is posterior or anterior. Again, Figure 8.25 shows the therapist placing his entire hand over the sacrum, his bottom hand is cupping the coccyx in a way that his fingers rest along the edge of the sacroiliac joints and his top hand

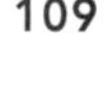

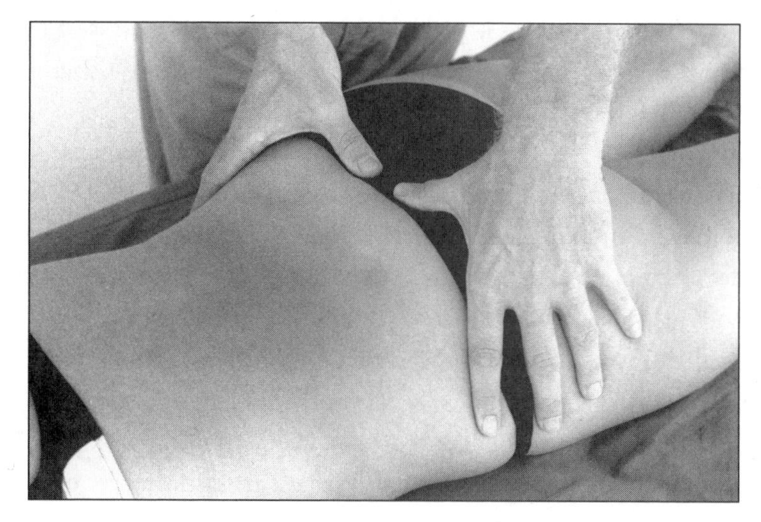

Figure 8.24

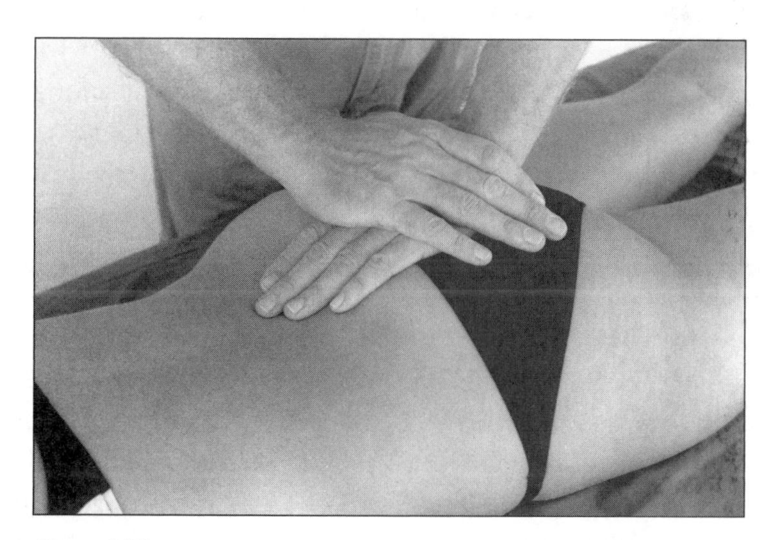

Figure 8.25

lies right on top of his bottom hand and is applying most of the compressional force. The reason you want to compress the sacrum and motion test it is to determine whether the anterior or posterior ligaments are fixed. If the sacrum does not respond to your pressure, then it means the posterior ligaments are tight. Alternately, if you compress the sacrum and it moves anteriorly, and as you very slowly release your pressure, the sacrum does not rebound into your hand, that is indicative of the anterior ligaments being fixed. This will guide your hands and eyes into other structures of the body that may be restricting the sacrum. If you determine from your motion testing that the posterior ligaments are indeed the ones that are causing the restriction in the sacrum or at least are at the epicenter of the restriction, then you can continue with the techniques and releases of the sacrum, low back, and the rotators. Even though what you are doing here is motion testing the sacrum to determine where the fixations are, just by motion testing you are also mobilizing the sacrum and its ligaments. As with all of the techniques, the sacrum needs to be compressed slowly so that you incrementally build up to the motion permitted, and as you release your hand, you do not release it all at once, but rather ounce by ounce you incrementally diminish your pressure so you can feel if the sacrum continues to move back with you into your hand.

The hand position in Figure 8.25 is the one you use to indirectly unwind the sacrum. Remember that you want to motion test three axes of rotation. First test flexion and extension around S-2. Say it moves easier into extension. From extension, you tip the sacrum right and left along its longitudinal axes. Now hold these two vectors firmly in place. Do not forget to follow the path of least resistance. Finally, side-bend the sacrum along the oblique axes and look for the direction of ease. Now you have stacked all three vectors. Maintain your pressure (up to several pounds) and wait for a release. This is the indirect style of unwinding, and the sacrum will generally respond well to indirect technique. If for any reason the client experiences pain during the technique, you must stop immediately. Pain is a contraindication.

There are many steps to this assessment. It is important to read this release in its entirety.

Sacroiliac Ligaments and Lumbar Fascia

This technique is particularly beneficial for clients with low back dysfunction and soft tissue problems of the pelvis. As you can see in Figure 8.26, the therapist has placed his elbow directly on the sacroiliac ligaments on the right hand side of the sacrum. You may like to begin at the inferior lateral angle of the sacrum on one side, and apply up to several pounds of compression into the sacrum with your elbow. Then very slowly glide over the fascia and the ligaments to the fifth lumbar and then stop. Repeat this process several times, both on the right- and left-hand side of the sacrum. There is also a tendency for the lumbar fascia to bunch up over the sacrum. This technique will give you more freedom in the three sacroiliac ligaments. Look at where the therapist's elbow is placed; he is directly on top of two of the sacroiliac ligaments, which are the horizontal and longitudinal posterior sacroiliac ligaments. If it causes pain, that is a contraindication, so it is important to stop. As an alternative with the clients that are very kyphotic, you can have the client prop herself up on her elbow, and this will assist you in creating a bit of a lumbar curve while you are working. You can also ask the client to lift her tailbone toward the ceiling while you are moving the fascia back down the sacrum toward its base next to the lumbars. Another excellent movement to ask for is to have her lengthen her femur bone down to the end of the table. This is very beneficial for mobilizing the various shorter ligaments around the L-5, S-1 junction, particularly to the iliolumbar ligaments.

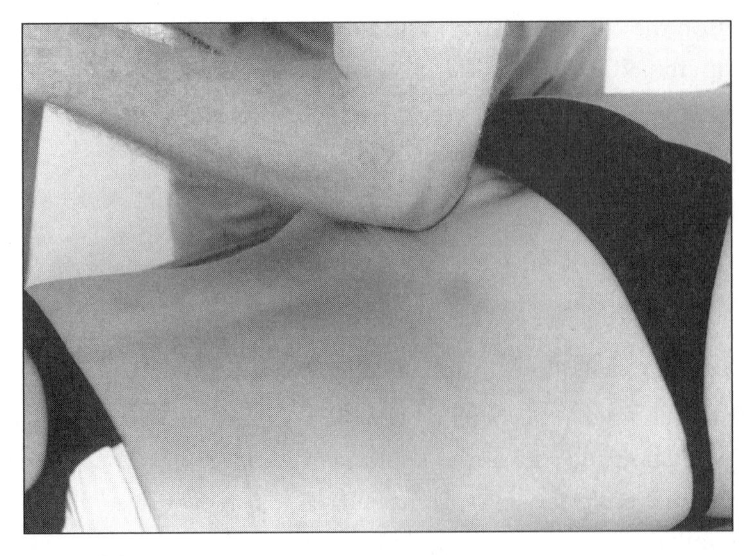

Figure 8.26

The Work: Sacroiliac Ligaments and Lumbar Fascia

Client Position: Prone

1. Face client's head and place elbow directly on the sacroiliac ligaments.

2. Begin at the inferior lateral angle of the sacrum and slowly glide over the fascia and the ligaments to the fifth lumbar vertebrae and then stop.

3. Repeat several times on both sides of the sacrum.

If this move causes increased pain, stop.

4. To increase the lumbar curve, have the client prop herself up on her elbows.

6. Movements to ask for are:

- Lift tailbone to the ceiling
- Lengthen the femur bone to the end of the table

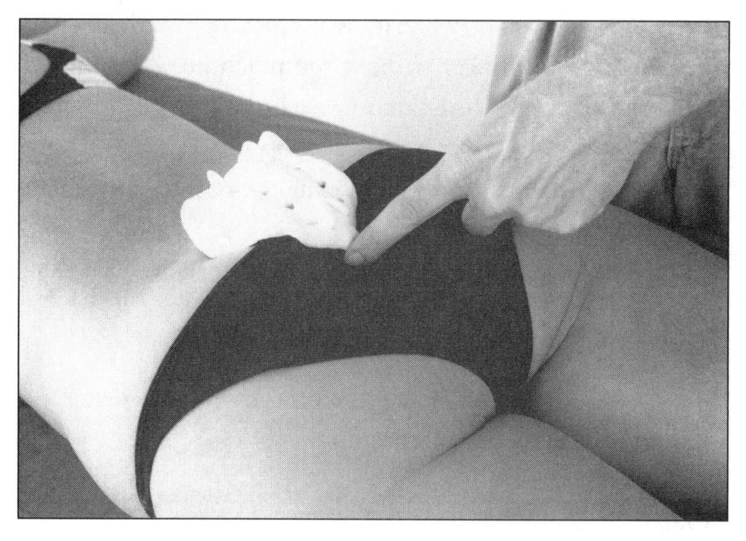

Figure 8.27

Coccygeal Ligaments

The coccyx has lateral ligaments on both its right- and left-hand sides, as well as anterior and posterior coccygeal ligaments. This technique can be very important for anyone who has ever had a fall on the tailbone and bruised it significantly. To start, you take your forefinger and palpate the coccyx very gently to determine its shape, its size, and its position. Sometimes the coccyx is bent anteriorly, but more often it is just bent to one side or the other. On the side it is bent toward, the ligaments will be much more dense and tight. Simply place your finger on the side of the coccyx that is tight or dense and gradually apply pressure as though you were forming a wedge between the coccyx and the sacrospinous ligament. Gradually you will feel the ligaments soften around the coccyx, and when this occurs, it is a good opportunity to motion test the coccyx with the tip of the finger. Put an ounce or two of pressure against the coccyx and see if you can get it to move back toward the midline. You can also mobilize the posterior ligaments if you feel that there is much more dense tissue on top of the coccyx. In this case, as shown in

Figure 8.27, what you may like to do is cross friction the ligament with the tip of your finger without too much pressure until you feel that the coccyx has begun to move a little. This is all you really need to do with the coccyx. You can have a very positive effect on the anterior ligaments just by mobilizing the posterior ligaments.

The Work: Coccygeal Ligaments

Client Position: Prone

1. Using forefinger, palpate the coccyx gently to determine its shape, size, and position.
2. Once the tight side is determined, apply several pounds of pressure as though trying to form a wedge between the coccyx and the sacrospinous ligament.
3. Wait for the ligaments to soften.
4. Once a softening is felt, motion test the coccyx with your fingertip.
5. Put an ounce or two of pressure into the coccyx and encourage it back to the midline.
6. Cross fiction the ligaments, if indicated.

Sacrum and L5-S1

This describes two techniques that are very valuable for releasing mechanical fixations of the L5-S1 junction. In Figure 8.28, the therapist takes his right hand and places the hypothenar eminence over the spinous process of the fifth lumbar. If you are not sure where spinous L5 is, you can palpate the superior edge of the crest of the ilium and draw a straight line back toward the midline of the spine. That will be approximately spinous L4. Then you only need to palpate one vertebra lower and you've got it. My compression, when the client is not experiencing any pain from it, can be up to 20 pounds of pressure directly on top of L5. You are compressing with two vectors. The first is an anterior compression toward the table, and the second is a slight superior compression. It is almost like a scooping motion in the sense that you want to follow or mimic the curvature of the lumbar vertebrae. The primary vector is an anterior compression. You will feel that the lumbars begin to give on the second or third exhalation of the client. Once you begin to feel this release occur, you gradually let go of your pressure. You can also, as you did before, prop the client up on her elbows, thus helping to reintroduce a lordosis into the lumbars.

Figure 8.29 shows the therapist holding a sacrum in the palm of his hand. This is a very delicate technique, especially if the client is holding any emotional or physical abuse issues in the pelvis. These issues afflict both men and women. Placing one's hand between the client's legs assumes that there is a great deal of safety and verbal permission to do so from the client. You should negotiate

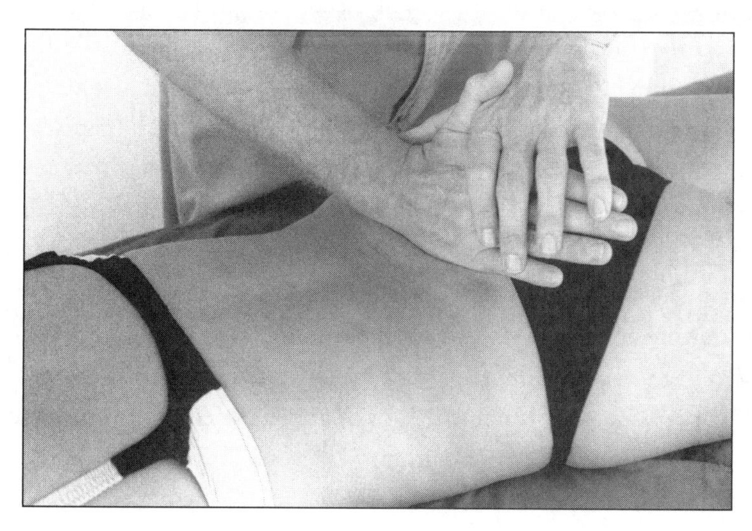

Figure 8.28

permission to do this, and if there is any hesitation, do not approach the client's sacrum in this way. With permission, place your hand in between the client's legs and allow the full weight of her pelvis to rest in your hand, with the sacrum located directly in your palm. If the client is not comfortable with this procedure, then either approach from the side or ask the client to lie prone and place your hand over their sacrum.

The simplest way to accomplish this decompression is to follow the respiratory pattern in such a way that when the client breathes in and out, the sacrum has a tendency to rock like a boat. There is a gentle rocking motion along a transverse axis that the sacrum makes during breathing. When you feel this motion begin to occur, you simply follow the sacrum with its micromovement toward the ceiling, that is, when the coccyx is moving anteriorly toward the ceiling and the base of the sacrum is coming into your hand. Then lift the sacrum as well as the whole pelvis, although your focus is just on the sacrum, with several pounds of pressure. Very gradually decompress the sacrum by tractioning it down toward the feet. Do this slowly. You may want to repeat it for two or three times until you get the hang of it. It is highly recommended to just hold the sacrum sometimes without any intention, but rather just letting the sacrum be in the palm of your hand and watch the involuntary motion that is induced by the respiratory diaphragm. Whatever is initiating the motion, you need only allow the motion for several minutes, and very often you will feel the sacrum push into the palm of your hand as though it is releasing from the inside of the pelvic floor. This has a very beneficial effect on the parasympathetic nervous system—molding the motion of the sacrum. It is also recommended that you use 2 or 3 inches of high density foam on top of your table if you plan to have the full weight of anyone's pelvis on your hand and wrist for more than a minute.

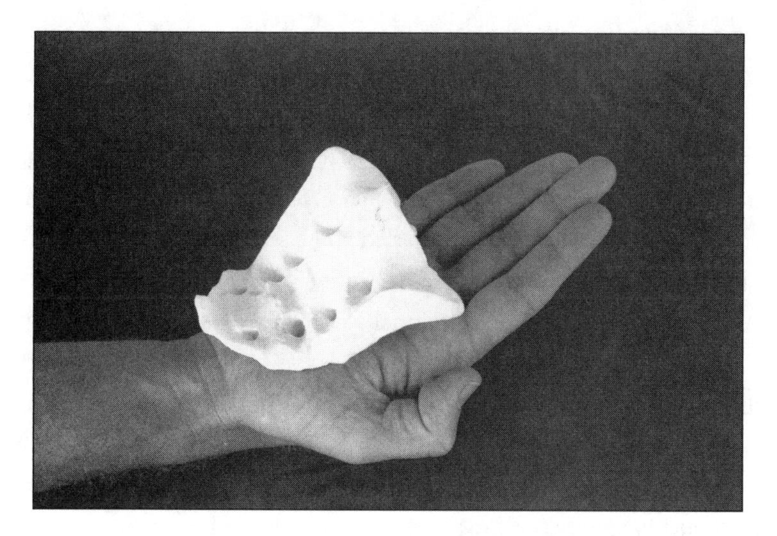

Figure 8.29

There are many steps to this assessment. It is important to read this release in its entirety.

Sacrotuberous Ligament

The release for the sacrotuberous ligament is an excellent follow-up to any work in the low back and/or the hamstrings, because the sacrotuberous ligament is really an extension of the hamstrings. There are numerous ways to release this ligament, but first you must know how to palpate it.

The ligament runs from the ischial tuberosity to the inferior lateral angle of the sacrum and is located one thumb's width above the tuberosity and one thumb's width medial to that point. First, place your thumb on the tuberosity and get a good feel for it. Then move your thumb into position one inch up and one inch medially from the tuberosity, and you will feel a very dense, thick ligamentous structure, which is the point to look for. Refer to Figure 8.30 for proper thumb or elbow placement. You may like to apply compression into the belly of the ligament and sometimes search the length of the ligament for thicker or tighter areas. You can also accomplish this technique bilaterally, and very often you will find one side is much tighter than the other. Begin to apply your compression with your thumb, or even your elbow, and you can build up to 10 pounds of pressure against that ligament. Figure 8.31 is an anatomical reference of the ligament in relationship to the pelvis. Have the client move her feet with dorsiflexion and plantar flexion as well as slowly lifting and tucking the tailbone while mobilizing the ligament. This will speed the process of the release and also carry the release much deeper into the fascial system. The trigger point for the sacrotuberous ligament is generally found right in the belly of it.

There is an alternative to this technique where you hook your thumb underneath the middle of the ligament and lift it out slightly. You may find this to be somewhat invasive for some clients, however, and may generally prefer to lean in on the ligament with your thumb or elbow while the client is making movement with her pelvis or legs. It cannot be stressed enough the importance of this one ligament and how often it is implicated in sacroiliac as well as sciatic types of pain referral patterns.

Along with checking the sacrotuberous ligament, it is recommended you go down into the hamstrings as a follow-up. As said in the anatomy of the sacrum earlier, there are two oblique axes of rotation that go from the right shoulder to left tuberosity, and from the left shoulder to right tuberosity. The sacrum moves around these axes when walking. Walking causes an alternating contraction and relaxation of each hamstring, which in turn pulls the sacrum along the oblique axes via the sacrotuberous ligament. The hamstring and sacrotuberous ligament act as one structure in this regard. This is why it is recommended to release the hamstrings following a release of the sacrotuberous ligament. The long head of the biceps femoris on the femur is frequently tight and very often overlooked when evaluating the hamstrings.

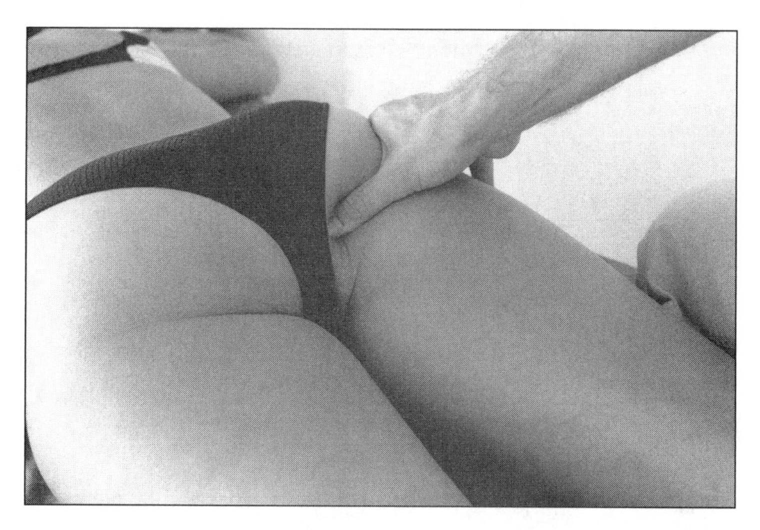

Figure 8.30

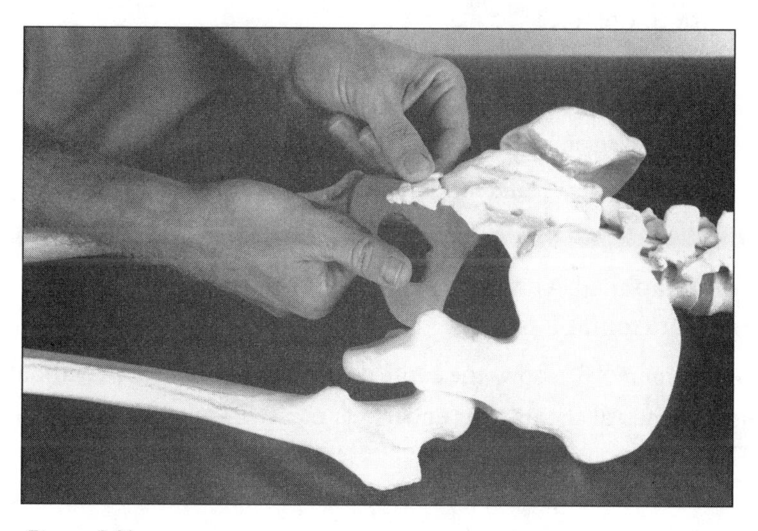

Figure 8.31

Work into the hamstrings as a follow-up, as the hamstrings and ligament act as one structure.

The Work: Sacrotuberous Ligament

Client Position: Prone

1. Place thumb or elbow on the tuberosity, move thumb one inch superior and one inch medial and a dense ligament should be felt.

2. Apply compression into the belly of the ligament, searching the length of the ligament for any tightness or thicker areas.

3. Movements to ask for are:

    - Plantar/Dorsiflexion of the foot
    - Slowly lift and tuck the tailbone

Topographical Anatomy of the Erector Spinae and Paraspinal Fascia

Note, Figure 8.32 shows the entire dorsal surface of the back without underwear. All clients wear underwear or a swimsuit when working. There are no exceptions.

When working with a client seated, you can also place both of your hands under the buttocks and palpate the position of the ischial tuberosities with the client's permission. Very often the client will not be thoroughly seated with equal amounts of weight on both tuberosities. This is a verbal cue you can give to the client when you feel her weight unevenly distributed. Let the right side of the body drop into your fingertips a little bit more, or vice versa. You

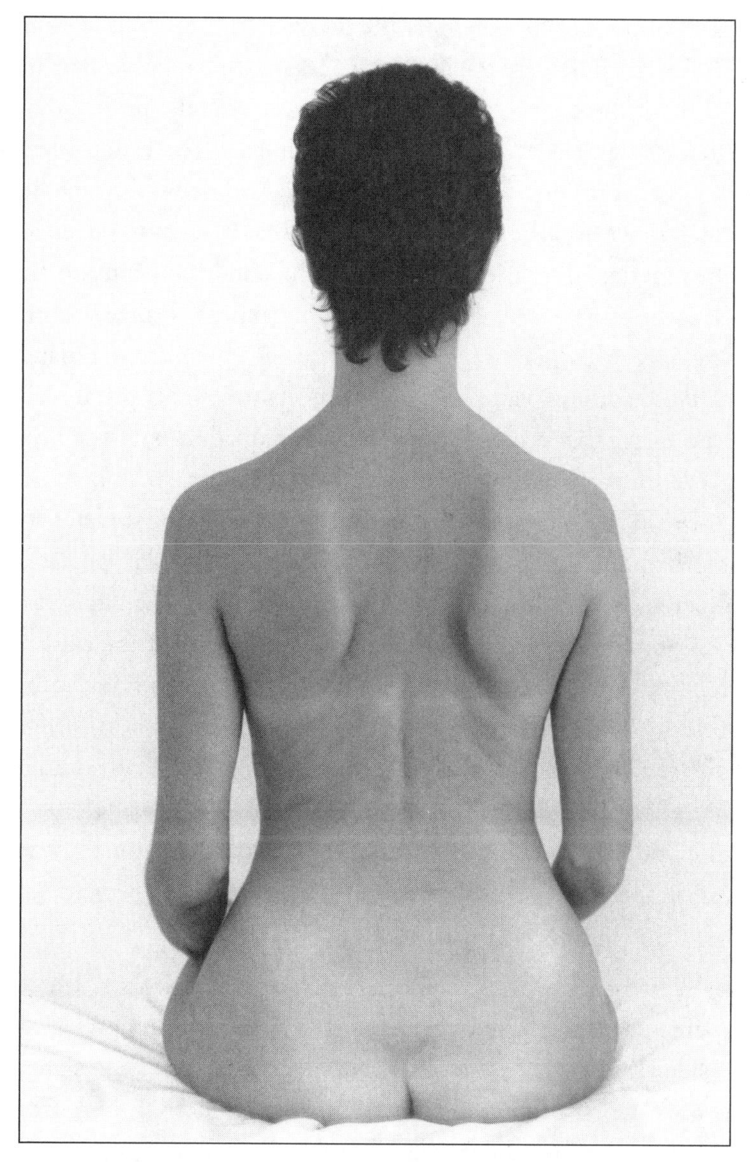

Figure 8.32

can also ask the client what that feels like once she shifts to an even balance and, surprisingly, she will very often report that she feels out of balance.

It is important to remember the two rules of thumb in working with the fascia that are the integrative fascia. Rule number one: the fascia over the erectors will tend to migrate laterally under stress. When it migrates laterally, the erectors shorten. You want to have an intention to move the paraspinal fascia from lateral to medial. Rule number two: the fascia shorten such that it needs to be moved from superior to inferior. It is valuable to stand the client up and look at the distribution of tissue around the spine. Visualize a central vertical axis that goes down the front of the spine, approximately where the coronal plane of the body meets the mid-sagittal plane of the body. This way you can look at the quadrants of the body and see the distribution of fascia and lack of symmetry. Then look at the side view of the client, specifically at her coronal plane and the distribution of the tissue between the anterior and posterior segments of the body. This will give you an idea of the amount of strain on the paraspinals and a relatively good look at the existing spinal curvature. Get a mental picture of the client's body before you begin work and do the same topographical analysis at the end of the session as a comparison. You are looking at the body and its orientation around a central vertical axis, and secondarily, looking at the body's orientation from front to back on the coronal plane.

Trapezius in Seated Position

This seated back work sequence is some of the best work. It does require you to take a bit of time to set up and do it properly. From the side view, you should look for a number of factors when a client sits down. First of all, you want her ankles to be slightly in front of her knees or just underneath. Figure 8.33 shows the client with her feet slightly ahead of her knees. If you were to look at a frontal view, you would see that her feet are no wider than her hips. The next step is to have the head of the femur parallel with the center of the knee, or ideally to have it slightly above the knee. The next thing you are looking for is that the client is sitting up straight

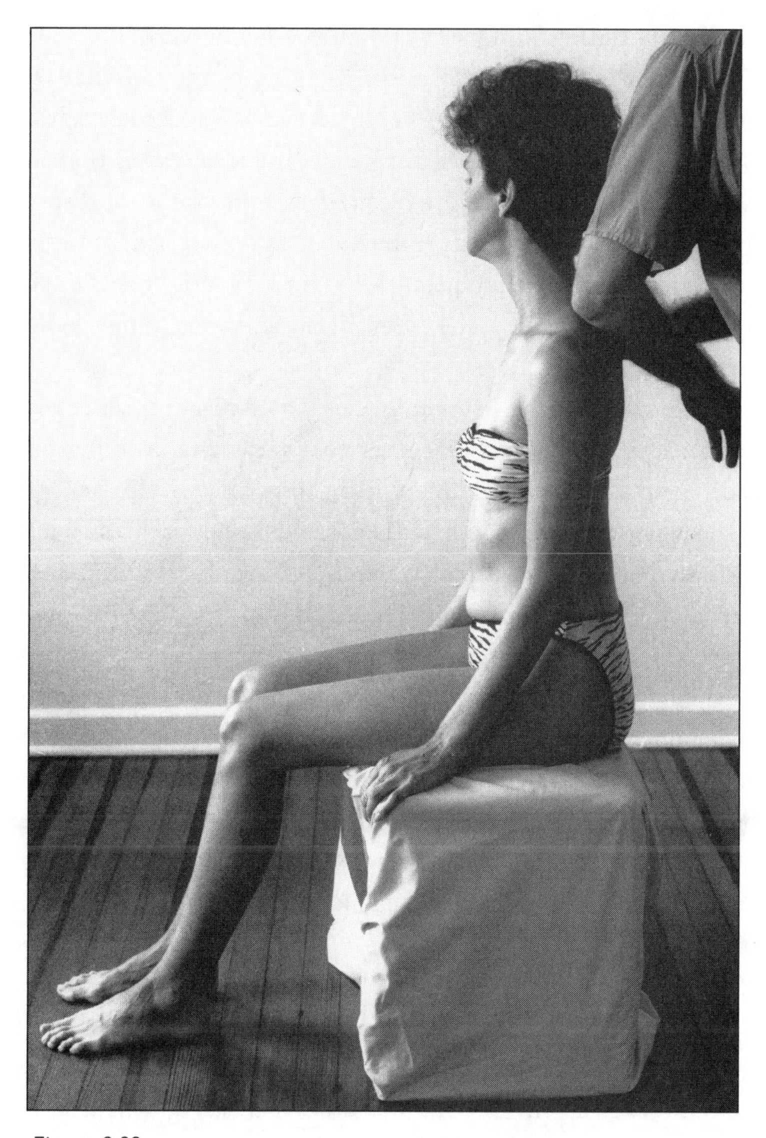

Figure 8.33

and not slumped. She can hold the lift while you are working. The shoulders and arms need to be hung loosely by the sides, and you can often touch the top of the client's head and ask her to lift her spine from the inside while you are working. This can be a stress position because so frequently when you begin work, the client collapses or in some way loses the integrity of the line that you are working. That means that her knees will splay out laterally or she will grip the bench with her hands. The idea here is that she is completely supported through her feet, tuberosities, and spine while you are working. That is the focus. The other benefit to this position is that if it is too painful or you touch a tight area or she gets genuinely fatigued, she will collapse and you cannot go any further until she gets a rest.

Once you have her lined up in this seated position, place your hand at the top of her thoracic vertebra and try to push her forward gently. While doing this, ask her to resist you with her feet. If she grasps the bench with her hands and pushes back, ask her to use only her feet. Once you have motion tested her spine and she knows what she is supposed to do, which is to give resistance with her feet, you can then begin working. Throughout the time that you are doing this seated back work, always keep scanning her body and giving her rest periods. You can often place your hands on the front and back of her diaphragm between units of work and ask her to breathe between your two hands. If you are working on the upper traps, when you take a break you will place your hand on the front and back of her thoracic outlet and likewise ask her to take a breath between your two hands.

When you work the trapezius, place your forearm over the superior edge of the trap and start to glide down and over the trap, moving toward the scapula. Repeat this two or three times on each side and gradually increase the pressure you are using each time. As your forearm continues to slide over the trap, you eventually get to the end of your forearm at the elbow where you securely hook the edge of the trap and its fascia. This is where you can apply more pressure as you are gliding over those superior and middle fibers of the trap that go over the rhomboids. One of the things that you can have the client do, as you can see in Figure 8.34, is to have her turn

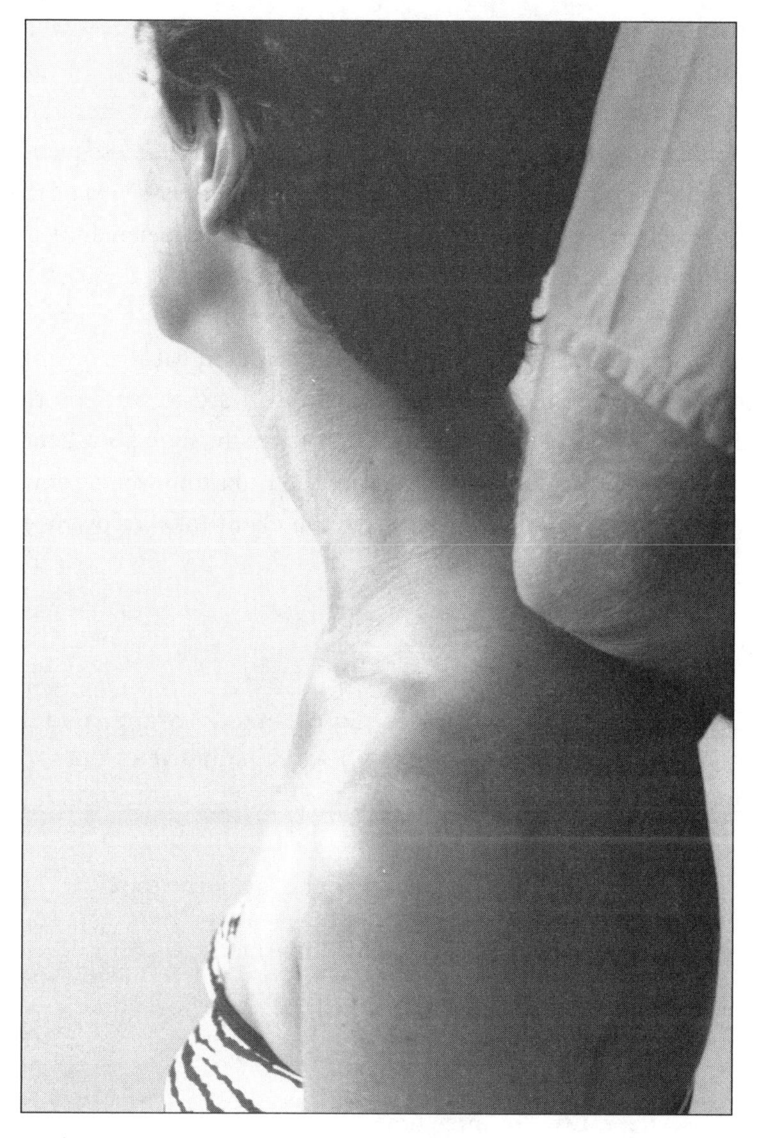

Figure 8.34

her head in the opposite direction from the side you are working on. As you work the trap, it is important that the client not collapse and that she continue to sit up straight as best she can, given the counter-pressure you are placing on the body. You can also cue her to lift the front of her spine up by pushing through her feet while working on her trapezius.

This is very effective work for anyone with chronic neck and shoulder problems and is an excellent way to finish any sequence of table work. It is really important that you get a sense of the placement of your elbow in the trapezius. Often times new students will compress the trapezius in a way that pushes the client off to one side. Rather, the pressure is down into the traps toward the bench, and it is essential that the client maintain balance on both of her sitting bones. It looks and feels awkward to work on the client while she is out of balance. Occasionally, slide both hands under her tuberosities and make sure she is putting weight down evenly on each of them. Then have the client take a slow, deep breath after each technique.

The Work: Trapezius Seated

Client Position: Seated, ankles slightly in front of the knees, feet no wider than the hips, hips slightly higher than the knee. Posture is a lengthening of the spine, resist with the feet, and arms loose at the sides.

1. Place forearm over the superior edge of the trap.

2. Spend a few seconds sinking into the tissues.

3. Start gliding down and over the trap moving toward the scapula.

4. Repeat two or three times.

5. Make sure pressure is appropriate and down toward the bench.

6. Encourage a deep breath after each technique.

7. Make sure the client does not collapse her posture by cuing her to lift the front of her spine by pushing with her feet.

Mid-Dorsal Fascia in Seated Position

Once you have finished working the trapezius and shoulder girdle, stand back from the client and ask her to drop her head and curl forward very slowly. Keep your eye on the individual vertebral segments as she rolls forward. Remember to have the client move in slow motion. As she curls forward, see which vertebrae are not moving independently with the vertebrae above and below that section. Have the client roll all the way forward until she cannot go any further. It may be wise at this point to have a pillow over her legs as this will feel a lot more comfortable when she is all the way forward. Ask the client to come back up into a seated position and have her once again roll forward, and this time make sure that she is also going forward from the hips and not just initiating the motion with her head and neck. It is as though there is a big beach ball in her lap, and she is just trying to roll her body over it. After repeating this several times, you will have a good idea of which vertebrae are hung up with the soft tissue and which are not. Then you can begin to work on the mid-dorsals.

Start off by taking your fists over the scapula and just move the tissue in toward the spine while she is holding a static position bent forward by 10 to 20 degrees as you show in Figure 8.35. Make two or three passes in the tissue and ask the client to sit back up and take a breath into her back. Then ask her to roll forward again and start another sequence of work with both your fists or one elbow, and this time you can work the tissue from superior to inferior by working down the lamina groove, down the posterior angle of the ribs, and/or down the edge of the scapula. All the while she is giving you resistance through her feet, and you are checking to

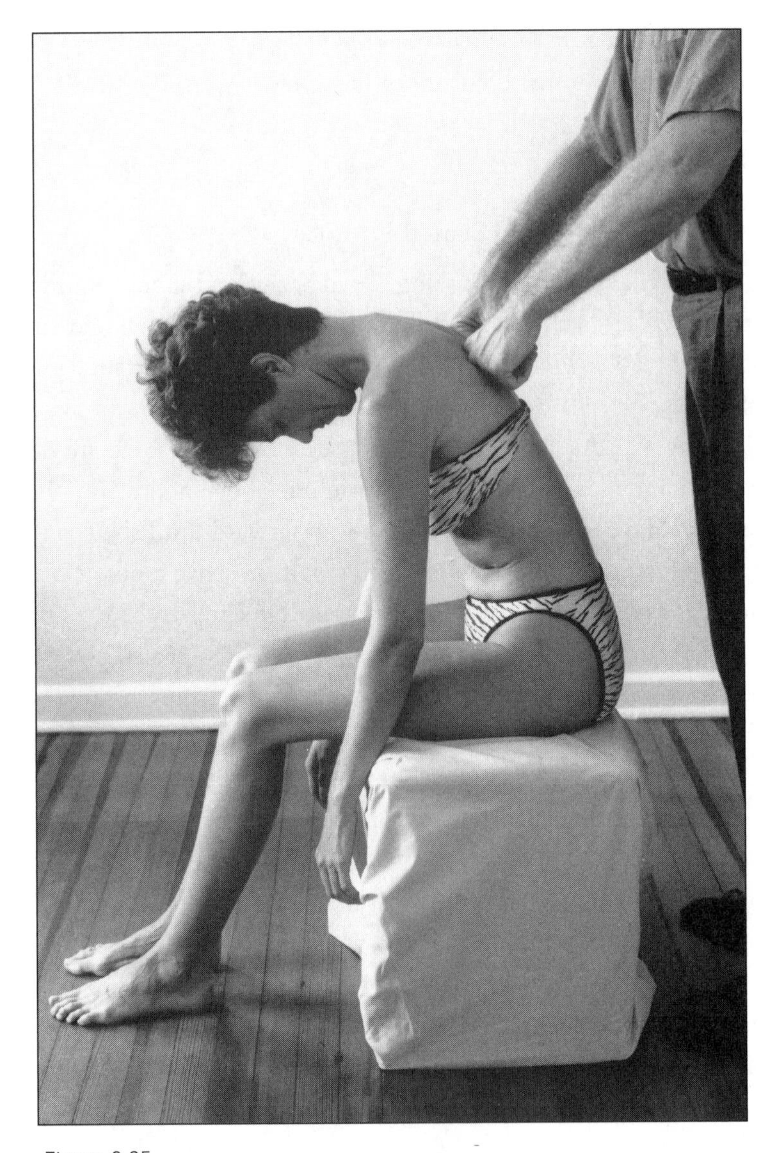

Figure 8.35

make sure that her arms and shoulders are hanging loosely and free. You also cue the client to let the forehead hang heavy or to move the forehead toward her knee. Many clients will then report a strain in the legs, and this is okay if it is not painful. Of course, the contraindication to this work is pain, especially along the spine or in the low back and hips. As an alternative, get hold of the tissue while she is seated upright, and begin to move the tissue toward the midline or down toward the sacrum as she begins to roll forward. It is almost like a dance. However, get familiar with this work from a static position before attempting to coordinate movement with the bodywork.

There are many things that you can do with the paraspinals in this position. Certain segments of the vertebrae have very dense pockets of tissue in the lamina groove or over the transverse processes, and you can cross fiber those segments. Whenever the client sits back up, you always place your hand over the area you worked on while your opposite hand is around the front on the ribs, and then you ask her to take a breath between your two hands. You also have the client reach out with your arms or hug herself. This opens up the latissimus and rhomboids for release work.

The Work: Mid-Dorsal Fascia

Client Position: Seated, ankles slightly in front of the knees, feet no wider than the hips, hips slightly higher than the knee. Posture is a lengthening of the spine, resist with the feet, and arms loose at the sides.

1. Ask client to drop her head and curl forward very slowly.

2. Move in slow motion.

3. As she curls forward, take fists over her scapula and move the tissues toward the spine.

4. Make two or three passes and ask the client to sit back up and breathe.

5. Ask her to roll forward again and work lamina, posterior aspect of the ribs, and the medial edge of the scapula.

6. Movements to ask for are:

   - Breath into the anterior and posterior ribs
   - Reach out with her arms
   - Hug herself

7. If the client feels uncomfortable at any time rolling forward, this work can be done in a static, upright position.

Lumbar Fascia in a Seated Position

This last segment of work is perhaps the easiest to do because the client is not offering any resistance with her feet. As mentioned earlier, it is recommended to place a pillow or two in the client's lap for support. These techniques should be performed with the client's ease in mind, especially since you are often applying a lot of pressure. The proper position of the client is demonstrated in Figure 8.36. Sometimes when a client bends forward, her knees will go lateral. At this point, have the client wrap her arms around and under her knees and hold them together. Use your elbow right along the lamina groove and the posterior angle of the ribs. You may recall all of the work described earlier on the three layers of thoracolumbar fascia and the quadratus lumborum. This is a good place and position to repeat that same sequence of work. The work in the middle septum between the erectors and the quadratus lumborum is especially valuable in this position. Clients that have had a laminectomy or fusion of their lumbar spine will love the way they feel after this work.

Remember that the client's face is out of view at this point, and it is not unusual for the client to get dizzy when she sits back up. Therefore, only do two or three passes in the tissue and have the

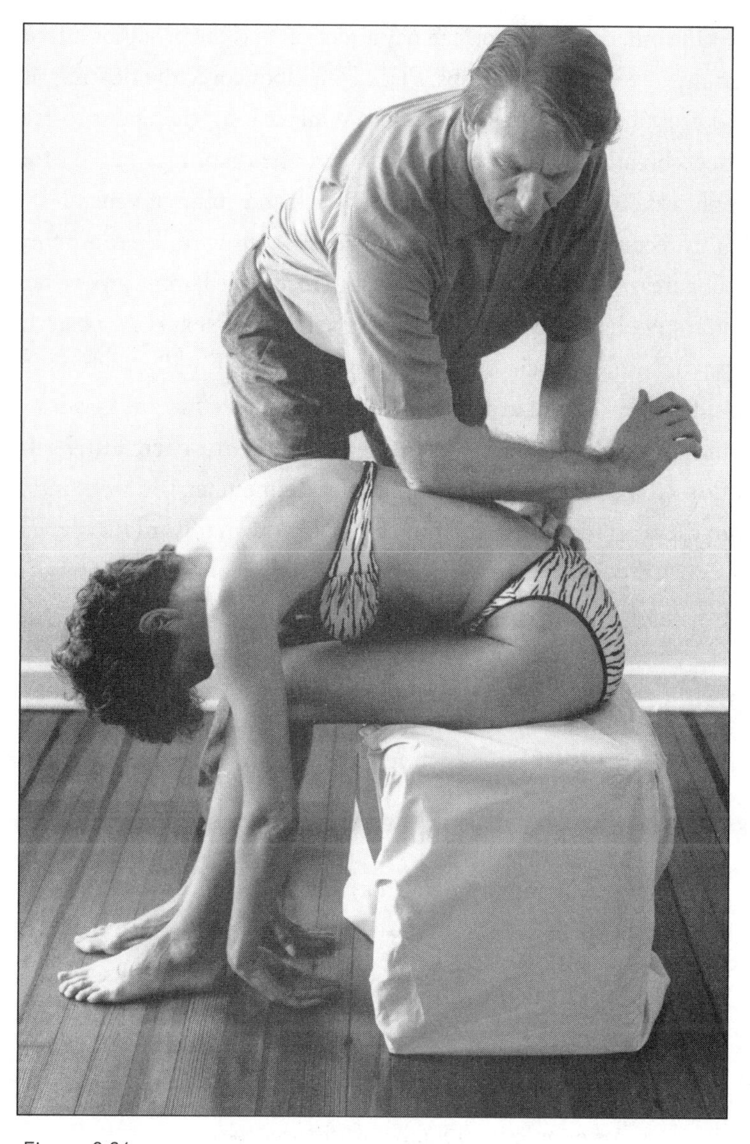

Figure 8.36

client sit back up. Then place a hand over her abdomen and low back, asking her to breathe into your hands. The elbow is the best tool for the low back. Continue the stretch all the way down over the sacrum and sacroilliac ligaments.

One other area that you can pay attention to is the posterior inferior serratus over the floating ribs. Place your elbow over the floating ribs and cross fiber the inferior serratus while asking the client to take a deep breath into the point of contact. The diaphragm is so often implicated in problems with the low back and spine in general. It is highly recommended to be a large focus in your work. There are three major areas to work in this position. The first is the lamina groove next to the spinous processes of the lumbar vertebrae. Next is the posterior layer of lumbar fascia over the erector spinae. Finally, there is the middle layer of lumbar fascia in between the erectors and quadratus lumborum. When working in this septum, have the client lean back a little so you do not knock her off balance. Remember, you are working into the septum toward the spine, as well as down toward the sacrum.

The Work: Lumbar Fascia

Client Position: Seated, ankles slightly in front of the knees, feet no wider than the hips, hips slightly higher than the knee. Posture is a lengthening of the spine, arms loose at the side. Can place a pillow in lap. Note: Client is not offering any resistance with the feet.

1. Have client wrap her arms around her knees in a bent over position.
2. Using elbow, mindfully work in these three major areas:
    - Lamina groove next to the spinous process of the lumbar vertebrae
    - Posterior layer of lumbar fascia over the erector spinae
3. Middle layer of lumbar fascia in-between the erectors and quadratus lumborum
4. Do not work so hard that the client gets knocked off balance.

5. Work medial toward the spine as well as down toward the sacrum.

6. Occasionally have client sit up and ask for breath with hands at the belly and low back, filling the space.

Paraspinal Fascia and the Thoracolumbar Fascia

This technique is some of the most important work you can do in myofascial release. The paraspinal fascia, and in particular the thoracolumbar fascia, are called the integrative fascia. Because of their proximity to the spine and the central nervous system, they need input during or at the end of each session of manual therapy.

In Figure 8.37, you can see that the therapist is at the head of the table and is using a broad contact with all of his fingertips. He is angling his fingertips toward the spine. You start a little more lateral and literally gather up or scoop up the fascia, and just move it toward the spine, being careful not to run over the spinous processes. You can do this all the way up and down the spine, just scooping and plowing tissue from lateral to medial. If you do this for 5 or 10 minutes, you will gradually see tone come into the erectors. It is okay to use your elbows or even your fist, as you can see in Figure 8.38. This photo, however, demonstrates the second principle of organization of the paraspinal fascia, and that is to move the tissue from superior to inferior. This will lift the trunk and lengthen the spine, all of which are very positive for those who have back pain. It shows the therapist with his fist working just lateral of the spinous processes of the vertebrae, with an equal amount of pressure on both sides of the back. It is important to remember to just do several inches at a time. Do not very often go the whole length of the spine because you are vitally interested in not overriding the respiratory or autonomic system with excessive contact.

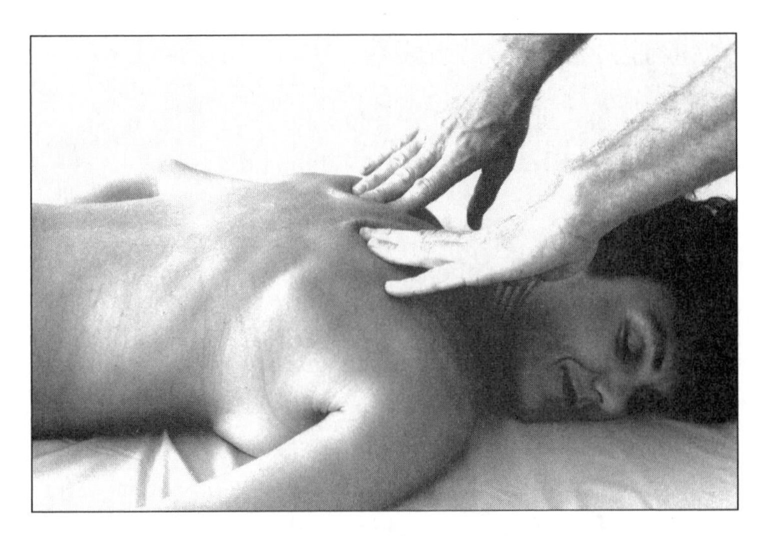

Figure 8.37

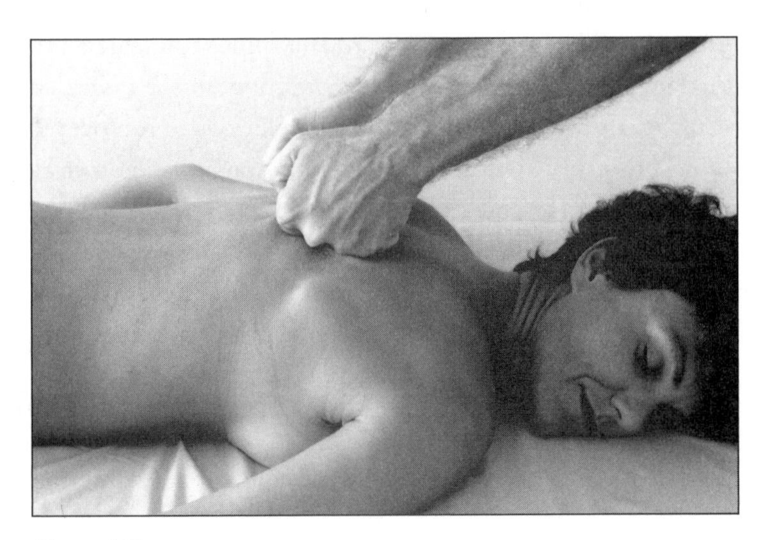

Figure 8.38

Figure 8.39 shows the broad contact and the bunching of the fascia as the therapist moves the tissue from lateral to medial. It is particularly demonstrative of the intention to move a broad plane of fascia. The pressure is deep, and the pressure is sustained. These movements are also short because they are gathering a lot of tissue and are not crossing over the spinous processes of the vertebrae. Figure 8.40 shows the therapist's thumb in the middle layer of lumbar fascia. What is recommended is to palpate the bulkiness of the erectors right at the top of the lumbars, around T12 and LI, and just lightly go over the erectors laterally until you get to the edge of the septum between them and the quadratus. Now imagine that you are trying to lift the erectors up by getting underneath them, and this gives you a very good entry into that middle layer. The action is to press your fingertips into the septum and form a wedge at the very top of the lumbars and then to very slowly glide down the septum toward the sacrum and even over the top of the sacrum slightly. This procedure can be repeated three to five times on each side of the lumbars. You may like to just do one side at a time and frequently ask the client to tuck her tailbone into the table and the reverse of that, to lift her tailbone slightly to the ceiling. Please remember not to ask for large movement here, just small movement up to maybe an inch in length. The movements are slow and smooth, not quick and jerky. This stretch, which organizes the middle layer, will also reflex into the anterior layer. The anterior layer of lumbar fascia is difficult to palpate because it merges at the aponeurosis of the internal and external obliques, close to the coronal plane of the body. So if you organize the posterior layer and the middle layer of lumbar fascia, and earlier in the treatment you have worked directly with the psoas, then you will have gotten all three layers of lumbar fascia. Consider this integrative work to be essential in myofascial release and something that you do with almost every client every time you see them, particularly at the end of a session.

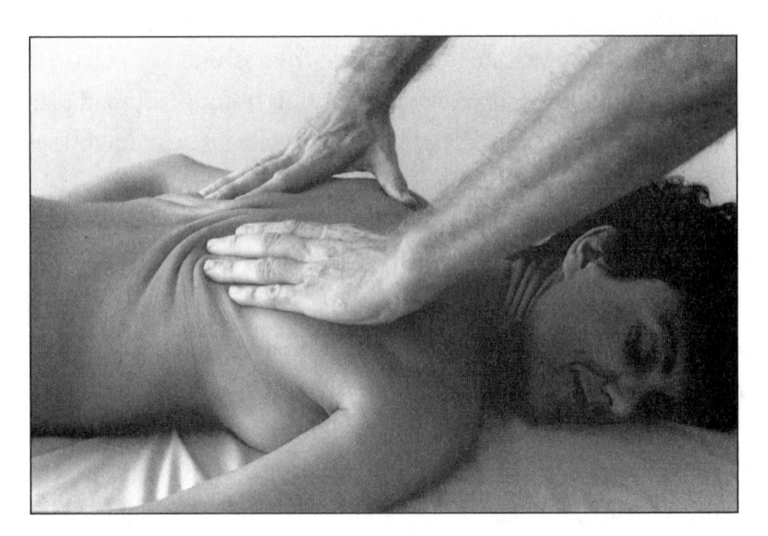

Figure 8.39

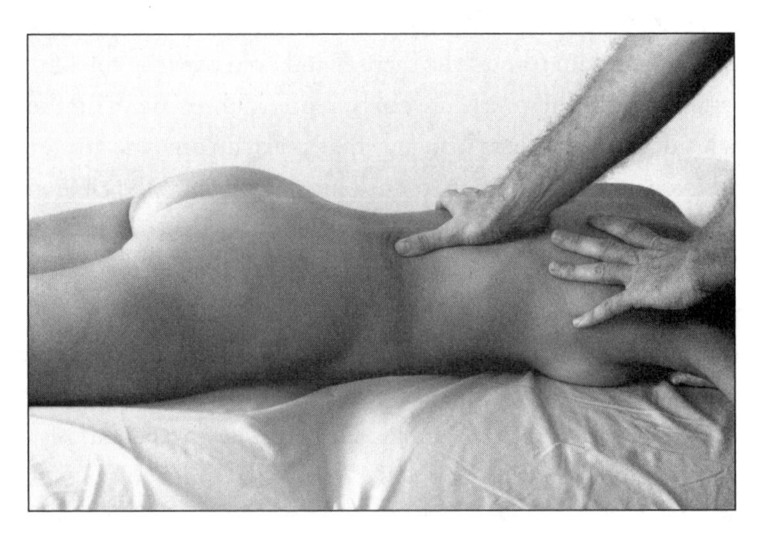

Figure 8.40

The Work: Paraspinal and Thoracolumbar Fascia

Client Position: Prone

Part 1

1. Stand at the head of the table and make broad contact with fingertips starting at the medial edges of the scapulae.

2. Angle direction of force medial or toward the spine.

3. Start laterally and scoop up the fascia and move it toward the spine.

4. Be careful not to run over the spinous processes.

5. Continue this all the way up and down the spine, making sure movements are only a few inches at a time.

6. Use fingertips, elbows, or fists.

Part 2

1. Move the tissues from superior to inferior using fists or elbows.

2. Use equal amounts of pressure.

3. Just do several inches at a time.

Part 3

1. Using thumb or fingertips at T12 and L1, move laterally until hands fall into the septum, the erectors, and quadratus lumborum.

2. Lift the erectors medially as if trying to get underneath them.

3. Run the septum gliding inferiorly toward the sacrum and even over the sacrum slightly.

4. Repeat three to five times on each side working one side at a time.

5. Movements to ask for are:
   - Tuck the tailbone
   - Lift the tailbone
   - Very small movements and very fluid

> Divide your work hour into three segments with a client. At the very beginning, work with the superficial fasciae of the body. During the middle period, for example the middle 20 minutes, go in and work the deep fasciae of the body. Finally, at the end of the session, spend at least 10 to 15 minutes, if not more, organizing the fascia. In this case, the lumbar fascia has three layers—the posterior, which goes from the sacrum to the cervicals and merges with the fascia of the capitus muscles. The middle layer goes from the transverse processes of the lumbar vertebrae to the crest of the ilium and twelfth rib. It forms a layer between the erectors and the quadratus lumborum. Finally, the anterior layer of lumbar fascia goes from the transverse processes of the lumbar vertebrae to the crest of the ilium and twelfth rib. It acts as a dividing layer between the quadratus lumborum and the psoas muscle.

The rule of thumb in working with the integrative fascia of the back is this: when the back loses its integrity by whatever means, orthopedic or organic, the fascia will migrate laterally and the erectors will shorten. This is a very simple rule of thumb, and its logic is something that has already applied to the front anterior surface of the body over the rectus abdominus. An overtight rectus will cause the trunk fasciae to migrate laterally. It is in this way that you can organize the fascia and thus bring a better organizational and energetic flow to the whole body by moving these fascia (and in this case speaking of the lumbar fasciae and other paraspinal fasciae), from lateral to medial.

CHAPTER 9

Releases of the Hip and Leg

Extensor Retinaculum and the Interosseous Membrane between the Tibia and Fibula

This is some of the most important release work in the lower leg. All injuries in the lower extremities will reflect in the ankle retinaculum. The way to begin this work is by placing the client in the side lying position (lateral recumbent) and, with your knuckles or fingers, place direct downward pressure on the lateral malleoli as shown in Figure 9.1. Slowly glide off the edge of the bone for an inch or so while maintaining pressure into the bone. Repeat this several times, asking the client for dorsiflexion and plantar flexion of the foot. It is important to maintain your compression into the ankle while the movement is happening. Only ask for movement occasionally and continue to loosen the tissue of the retinaculum for several minutes. You can move several inches superior to the ankle and inferior as well. In addition, you can spread the medial malleoli with the pads of your fingertips, like a deep bear claw, to treat the opposite side. Move back and forth between the two. It is important to take a break every minute or so and ask the client to take a breath or to just relax if she experiences a lot of sensation with this work. Start on the midline of the ankle and work away from the midline. It can be done for 10 to 15 minutes on each ankle. As an alternative, you can place the client in supine and work both sides of the ankle at once. Occasionally move your attention to the foot as well.

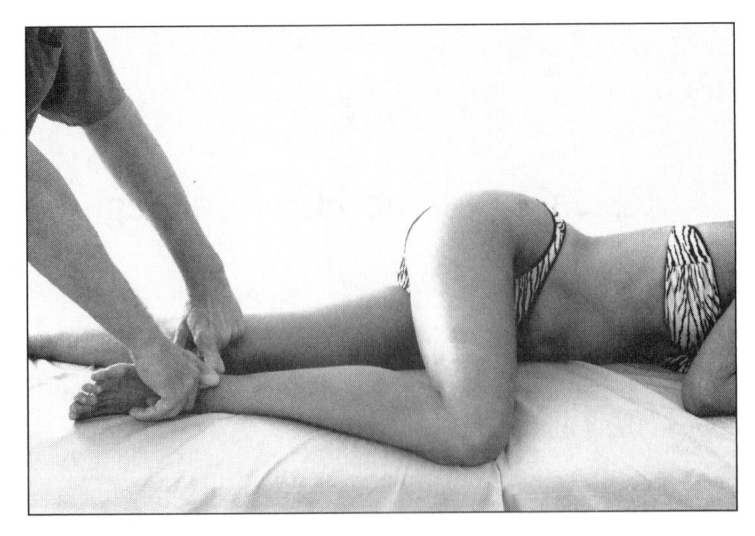

Figure 9.1

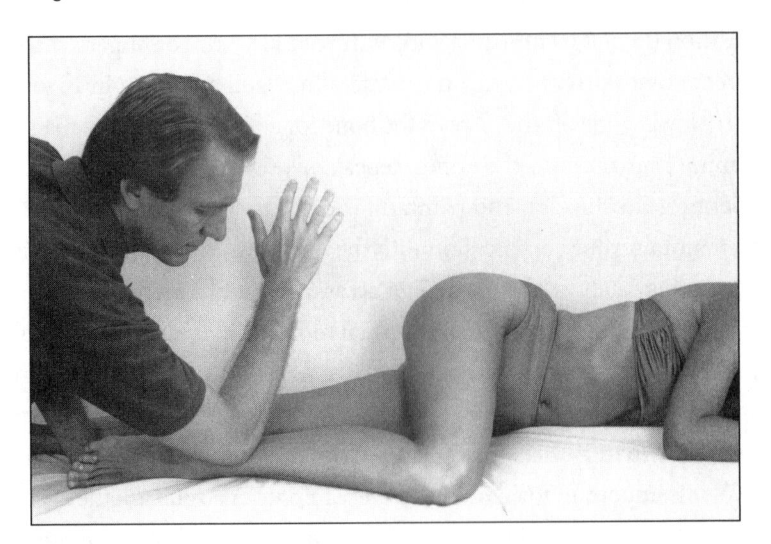

Figure 9.2

Figure 9.2 shows the therapist using the point of his elbow and moving up the extensor digitorum longus compartment. This is located right between the tibialis anterior, which lies along the tibia, and the fibularis muscles, which lie along the fibula. Start just above the retinaculum using the point of your elbow, fingertip, or knuckle. Apply slow, deep pressure at an angle toward the interosseous membrane until you contact the tight layer of tissue. At this point, maintain your pressure and start to move superiorly toward the knee. Go slowly, and only move several inches at a time, and occasionally ask for dorsiflexion and plantar flexion of the foot. If you find a very tight area, you can roll your elbow back and forth over it. It is important to keep an eye on the client's respiratory mechanism and occasionally ask her to take a deep breath if you see that she is holding her breath. Move several inches at a time, take a break, and move slowly and incrementally. You can also ask the client to tuck her tailbone forward and back as an additional movement request that is done to facilitate freedom in the deep fascia of the leg and pelvis. You do not have to cover the whole length of the extensor compartment in order to facilitate a release. Usually the area that is the most stuck is just superior to the malleoli. This is where the deep and superficial fascia of the body merge, and is therefore an area for potential restriction. This work is excellent for anyone with ankle and knee problems as well as back problems.

The Work: Extensor Retinaculum

Client Position: Side lying, with top knee flexed at 45° (lateral recumbent) or supine

1. Use knuckles or fingers.

2. If working side lying, place downward pressure into both sides of the lateral malleoli, slowly gliding off the edge of the bone.

3. If working supine, place downward pressure starting at the midline of the ankle and working laterally.

4. Repeat several times. This work can be done for 10 to 15 minutes per ankle.

5. Take a break every minute or so, asking the client to take a breath.

6. Occasionally ask the client for dorsiflexion and plantar flexion of the foot.

The Work: Interosseous Membrane

Client Position: Side lying, with top knee flexed at 45° (lateral recumbent)

1. Place an elbow just above the retinaculum.

2. Apply slow, deep pressure in toward the membrane until contacting the stuck layer.

3. Move superiorly toward the knee, moving slowly asking for dorsiflexion and plantar flexion.

4. Friction if necessary.

5. Client can tuck tailbone as an additional movement.

> Sometimes the movements clients attempt to make are too big. Break the dorsiflexion down in to three smaller movements: toe up, foot up, press through heel.

Achilles Tendon

Figure 9.3 shows the therapist's knuckle being used to stretch the aponeurosis of the heel cord and gastrocnemius. His direction of pressure is moving into the heel cord to the point of restriction and then down toward the foot just an inch or two at a time. Notice that his opposite hand is on the same foot, and he is plantar flexing and dorsiflexing the ankle in order to assist the release through the heel cord. Another area of potential restriction is on either side of the tendon, so it is good to go into the side of the heel cord and do the same stretch down toward the ankle. Notice in the photo that he is supporting the leg with his thigh. You can also do this with a pillow or some other type of support.

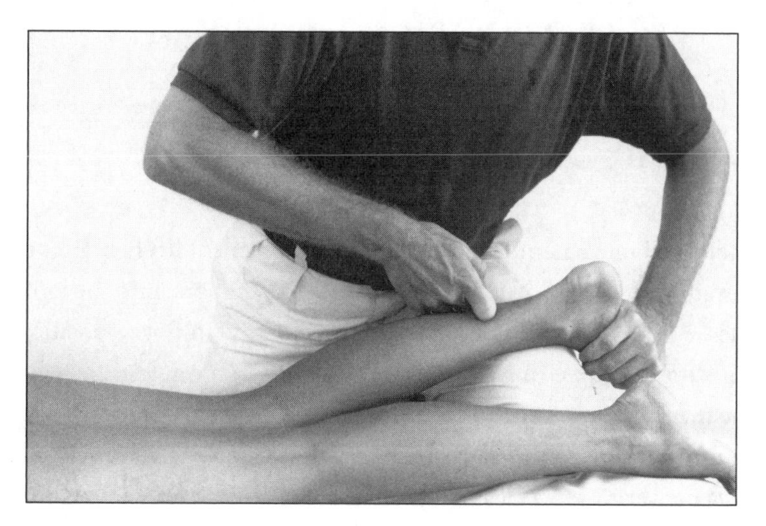

Figure 9.3

Next, in Figure 9.4, the therapist is using the point of his elbow on the heel cord. Here you have a tendency to roll back and forth on the fascia that is particularly thick and tough. You make sure that the client has the foot extended beyond the edge of the table, so that when you ask for foot flexion, her feet don't bump into the edge of the table. This photo shows the leg unsupported; however, in many cases you will need to place some type of support under the leg because of pressure being used into the heel cord with your elbow. The posterior fascia is continuous with the sacrum. An

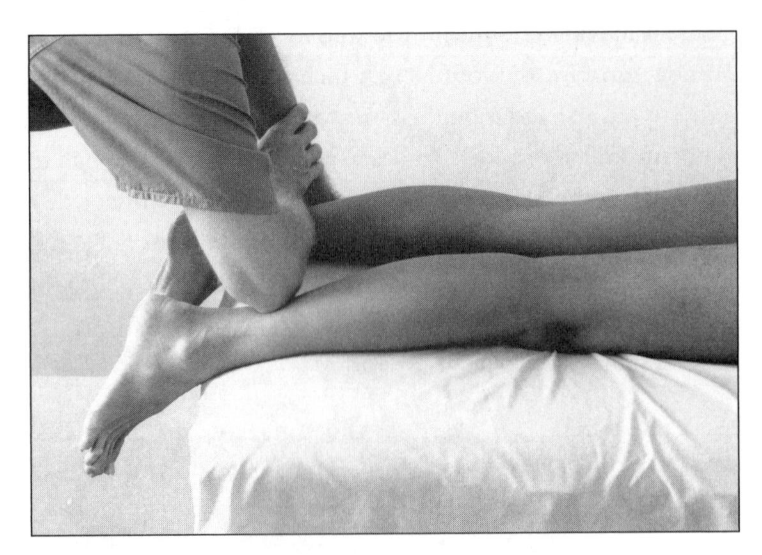

Figure 9.4

additional movement to ask for is to have the client lift her tailbone toward the ceiling and alternately to tuck her tailbone into the table. Please notice that in both photos, the client is in prone position, with the foot free to go through a range of motion. The area that the therapist is working on is several inches in length, and it is okay to move up into the gastrocnemius or even lower down over the fascia covering the calcaneous.

The Work: Achilles Tendon

Client Position: Prone, with feet hanging over end of table

1. Use elbow or knuckle to move inferiorly into heel cord moving inferiorly an inch or so at a time.

2. Use opposite hand to dorsiflex and plantar flex the foot to help facilitate the release, or ask the client to make the movement.

3. Using 15 to 20 pounds of pressure, use elbow to travel

from the heel cord up into the gastrocnemius making sure the foot has full freedom of movement.

4. Friction the medial and lateral aspects of the tendon if needed. You can displace the tendon in either direction to have better access.

5. Always be mindful of the rule of stop.

Plantaris and Gastrocnemius Muscles

Before beginning these techniques, it would be valuable to look in your anatomy books and get a good image of this muscle and long tendon. It originates on the lateral epicondyle of the femur, crosses the knee and goes down the medial edge of the soleus and Achilles tendon. The therapist's finger actually points to the trigger point and the entry spot for the release in Figure 9.5. You must weave your way around the tendons of the hamstrings. Do this with the knee flexed at a 45° angle. The photo shows the knee at an oblique angle so you could see precisely where the therapist goes in. When you get around the hamstrings, press your finger straight down toward the table and the patella. Bump right into the trigger point. It will naturally feel hard since it is on the bone. Ask the client if she feels any tenderness. You may want to move your finger in a small circle around the epicondyle until you find the tenderness. The skill with this technique is to use your opposite hand to plantar flex the foot. Apply one pound of pressure, and when the trigger point releases, you will naturally feel the foot plantar flex. At that point, you can add a bit more pressure and facilitate a good stretch. This procedure should only take 30 to 60 seconds and is wonderful for tight knees, ankles, and heel cords.

Next is a stretch for the fascia of the gastronemius. As you can see in Figure 9.6, the therapist is using his thumb to hold the fascia while plantar flexing and dorsiflexing the foot. The pressure is deep, and he

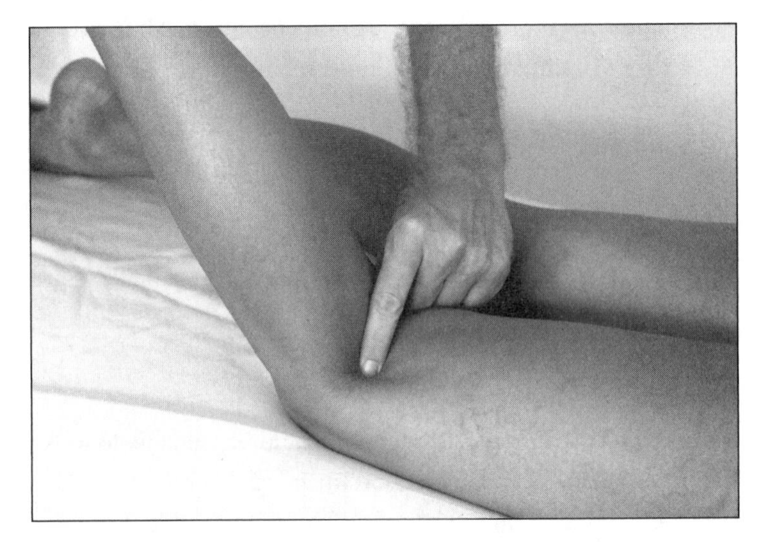

Figure 9.5

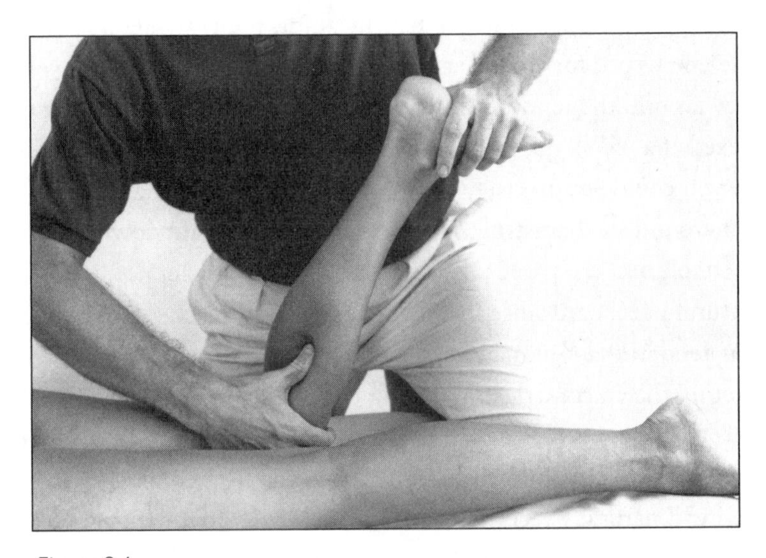

Figure 9.6

is moving toward the feet several inches at a time. You may frequently take a break and ask the client to take a breath. This is an important part of the technique. Some lower legs are going to be too muscular for your thumbs. Another option is to allow the feet to hang off the end of the table, with enough room for the client to freely move her foot, and use your elbow to pin the fascia while asking for movement.

> It is conscious breathing that allows soft tissue to integrate with the nervous system. It is a tendency among inexperienced therapists to overuse deep tissue work. This does not resolve the problem but exacerbates the trauma. A client after a session may look disoriented from overwork, and it is a mistake to think that this represents relaxation or better tone. You do not have to work as hard. When you take a break, keep scanning the client's body and look for other clues that the nervous system is giving you about integrating your work. You want to watch not only the breath, but also the facial expression, skin color tone, tight jaw with overtone in the masseter and temporalis muscle, sweaty palms and feet, and finally the eyes. Remember, with computers, you have to stop inputting every now and then because that little clock or hourglass pops up and tells you that the software and hardware are integrating. You cannot move forward until this process is complete. A body will do this by taking a deep breath and other ways as well, so keep your eyes open.

The Work: Plantaris

Client Position: Prone

1. Place finger medial to the hamstrings on the lateral side of the knee.

2. Press straight down until contact is made with the lateral epicondyle of the femur.

3. Use about 1 pound of pressure.

4. Once contact is made, use opposite hand to plantar flex the foot.

The Work: Gastrocnemius

Client Position: Prone

1. Place thumb into the gastrocnemius searching for tight tissue.

2. With appropriate contact, dorsiflex and plantar flex the client's foot.

3. Take frequent breaks and ask for breath.

4. This can also be done using an elbow with the knee in extension while asking for movement.

Medial Hamstrings

This release is a simple stretch of the medial hamstrings. Start by placing your elbow into the belly of the muscles and slowly move up toward the ischial tuberosity. The movements to ask for are pressing the knee into the table, lifting the foot toward the ceiling, dorsiflexing and plantar flexing the foot, and lifting and tucking the tailbone. The foot flexing and the tailbone movement are especially good with this technique. The starting point for most of these areas is with the point of your elbow, and when you open up the angle of your elbow, you will give yourself a much larger working area. You can see in Figure 9.7 that the therapist's arm is almost completely flexed. Once you start your glide up toward the tuberosity, open your elbow up and use a broader elbow/forearm surface. This causes less pain and also affects a much broader plane of fascia. It is not recommended to go the whole length of the muscle. The way to check this is to test the range of motion and see if it is greater, to see if the motion itself appears to be easier, or to ask the client if she feels a release. If you move slowly enough into the tissue as the biochemical and electrical changes begin

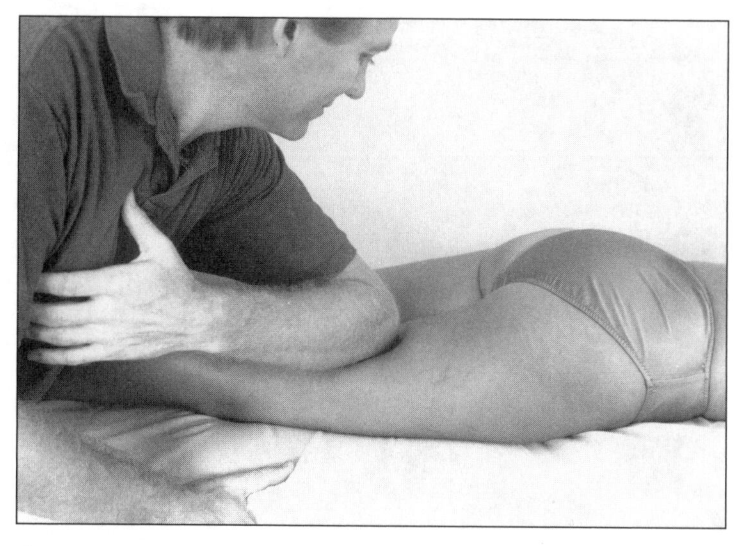

Figure 9.7

to take place, you can feel the changes in the elastic and buoyant quality of the tissue. There may not be a need to continue once you sense this happening.

The Work: Medial Hamstrings

Client Position: Prone

1. Place elbow into belly of the muscle and move slowly toward the ischial tuberosity.

2. Use broader pressure when working in larger planes of fascia.

3. Movements to ask for:

    - Press knee into table
    - Dorsiflex and plantar flex foot
    - Lift and tuck tailbone

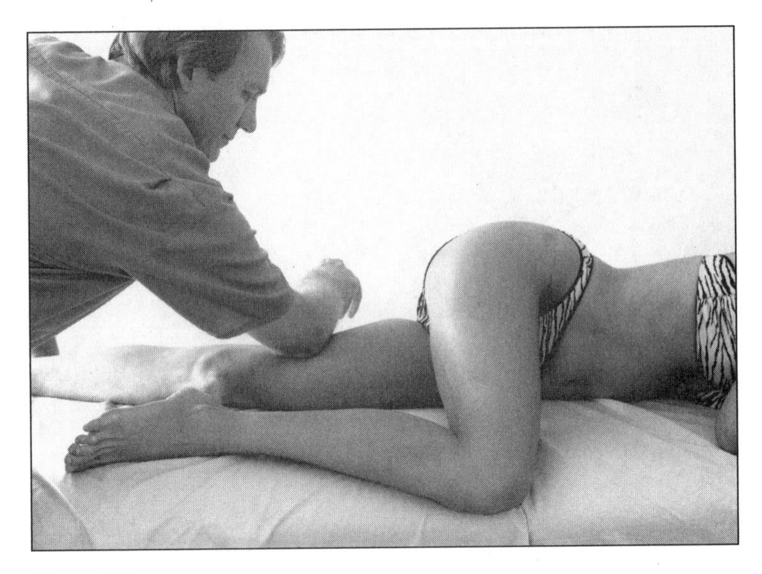

Figure 9.8

Adductor Magnus and Its Attachments on the Ramus of the Ischium

Figure 9.8 shows the starting position on the adductor magnus. You want to make sure that you position yourself in front of the client, while your vector is from front to back. The next step is to place the broad surface of your forearm on top of the adductor several inches above the knee.

Start by applying a very slow and incrementally deeper pressure down into the adductor until you feel any tension or tight areas. Slowly move your forearm posteriorly, taking up all the slack in the skin and superficial fascia of the leg. As your forearm glides back over the adductor magnus, fall into the septum between the adductor and the hamstring. Pause there and ask for movement. The movement is tucking the tailbone forward or backward, or you can ask for a heel stretch or knee flexion. Once you are in the septum and have asked for those motions sequentially, then very slowly glide over the top of the medial hamstring. One of the consistent problems of the lower leg is that the fascia over the hamstrings migrates medially over on top of the adductors. You can repeat this procedure two or three times over the same area until you feel that the tissue has released or softened. Then you can move on closer to the ramus of the ischium and repeat the same procedure.

> Notice in Figure 9.8 that the opposite leg of the client is stretched at a 45° angle. For the sake of this photograph, do not use any support for the knee; however, in practice, the knee should always be supported when doing this technique or any side lying technique.

The next part of this technique is to work on the ramus of the ischium. To start this technique, place the whole palm of your hand on top of the adductor magnus, as shown in Figure 9.9, and very slowly melt your way down into the muscle. Very slowly bring your fingers into contact with the ischial tuberosity of the leg. When your finger or fingertips are in contact with the tuberosity, you can palpate around the tuberosity and feel the attachments of the hamstrings. This technique is very simple because all you need to do is come in contact with the bone and put a very slight pressure, maybe several ounces to no more than a pound or two, up against the bone and gently cross-friction. You will feel the fascia melt and soften. After palpating around the tuberosity, remove your fingers and ask the client if she is comfortable before proceeding. Then place your hand palm down once again, and this time move forward of the tuberosity onto the inferior ramus. Your fingertips will come into contact with the inferior ramus, similar to the tuberosity. Again, you make a very slight friction motion back and forth with your fingertip just an inch at a time while pressing into the bone. Ask the client to take a breath into the point of contact several times.

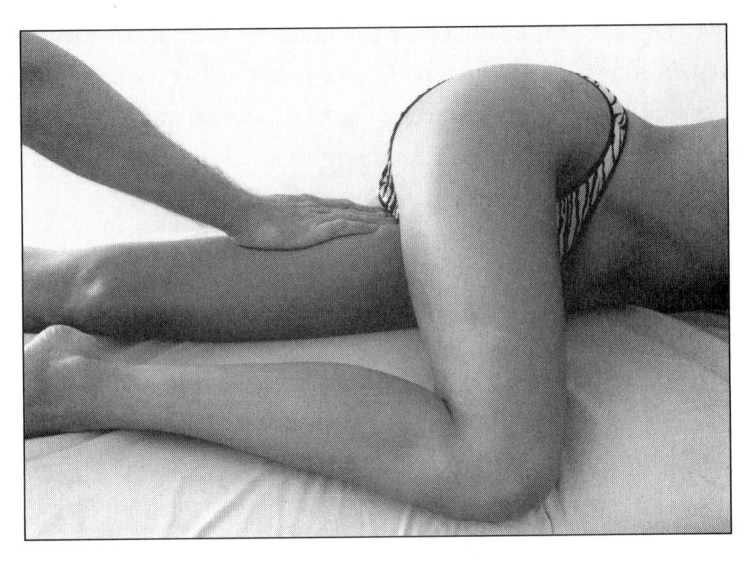

Figure 9.9

Repeat this procedure two or three times on different sections of the ramus, making sure that you give the client a break in between.

The Work: Adductor Magnus

Client Position: Side lying, with top knee flexed at 45° (lateral recumbent)

1. Facing client's head, working in front of the client's body, apply very slow but deep pressure into the adductor magnus.

2. Apply slow deep pressure moving back and forth looking for tension and tightness.

3. Movements to ask for are:

    - Tuck tailbone forward and backward
    - Stretch heel
    - Flex knee

The Work: Ramus of the Ischium

Client Position: Side lying, with top knee flexed at 45° (lateral recumbent)

1. Place whole palm on the adductors and apply slow deep pressure.

2. Glide up the midline of the leg making contact with the ramus.

3. Use a gentle scooping or sweeping movement waiting for fascia to soften.

4. In addition, move posteriorly to work the ischial tuberosity where the hamstrings attach.

Piriformis and Biceps Femoris Muscles

Remember that the piriformis is attached to the anterior surface of the sacrum and to the greater trochanter of the femur. Your elbow placement is midway between these two points, shown in Figure 9.10. Take your free hand and flex the client's knee to a 45° angle. Before applying too much pressure into the piriformis, motion test the femur by gently rotating the leg laterally and medially. This should help the placement of your elbow, as you will feel the piriformis and the rotator compartment contract. Slowly begin to apply pressure into the piriformis, and at the same time, slowly rotate the leg back and forth with your opposite hand. Even better, have the client move her own leg to avoid putting unnecessary pressure on the knee. Then ask for movement by having the client lift her tailbone up to the ceiling and then tuck it toward the table. She does not need to do the leg rotation and tailbone lift at the same time. Some of the other options you have with the piriformis are to glide your elbow to the trochanter and to work the fascia off

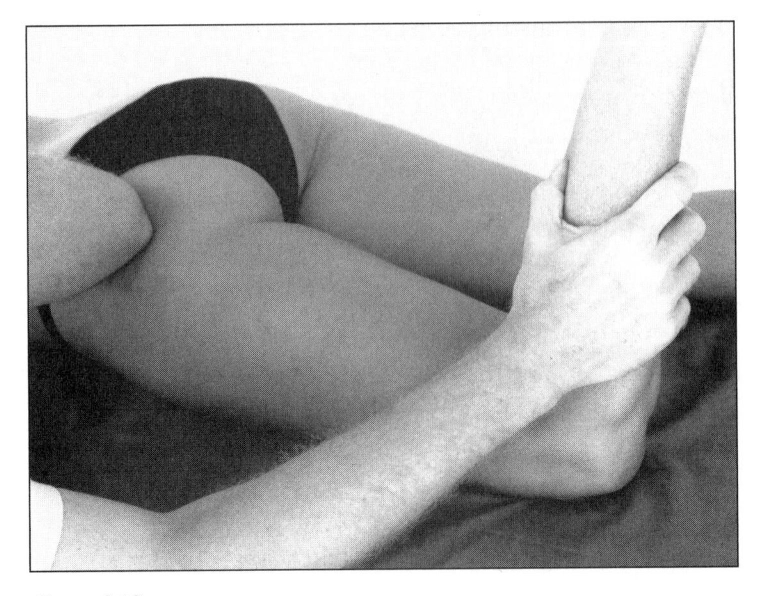

Figure 9.10

of the trochanter. This is where all of the rotators attach, and it is particularly beneficial to have your free hand rotating the femur. You will feel your elbow sink in to a much deeper place around the femur. You can also keep the leg extended as an option and ask the client to rotate her leg.

It is not recommended to do this technique with someone who has acute sciatic pain.

In Figure 9.11, the therapist is moving on to work the biceps femoris. It has a long attachment along the body of the femur and is easily accessed via the septum between the hamstrings and the IT band. Start with your pressure directly on the bone, several inches below the trochanter. Like some of the earlier techniques, just go several inches at a time. At the ischial tuberosity,

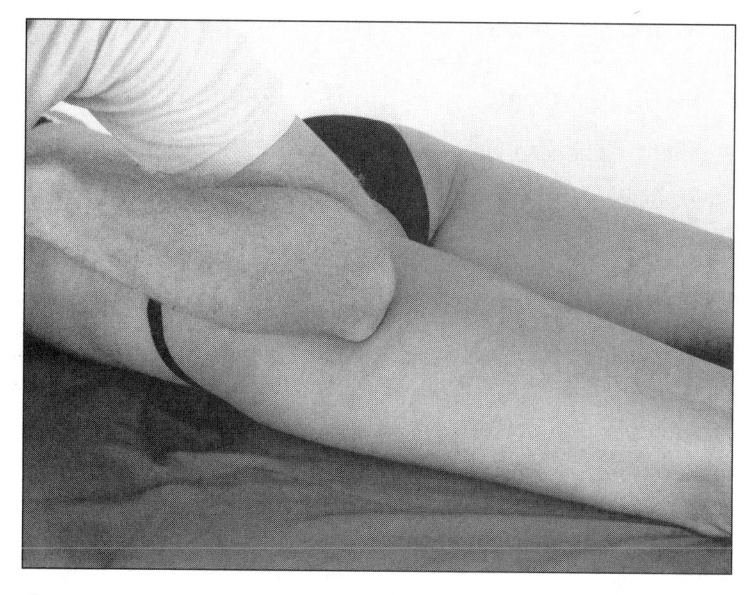

Figure 9.11

you can muscle test by asking for knee flexion to make sure you are medial enough. This is one technique where you may want to ask for a lot of movement. You can alternately ask the client to lift her foot up, to press her knee into the table, to dorsiflex or plantar flex her foot, and to lift and tuck her tailbone. The photo shows the therapist with his back to the client's face, so he needs to remember to stop, move around, and take a look at her diaphragm and facial expression. The closer you get to the knee, the more intense the sensation can become. It is important to go slow and easy as you approach the knee. Use this technique on every client who has had knee replacement surgery or any orthopedic injury to his or her knee, especially the short head of the biceps femoris.

The Work: Piriformis

Client Position: Prone

Gently place an elbow into the piriformis searching for tight tissue or trigger points.

Check placement by motion testing the femur using medial/lateral rotation.

Gradually increase pressure while continuing to rotate the femur.

A better option is to ask the client to rotate the femur on her own to avoid over stretching.

Another movement to ask for is a pelvic tilt.

The Work: Biceps Femoris

Client Position: Prone

1. Place elbow directly on the bone several inches below trochanter moving medially into the septum between the IT band and the bicep femoris.

2. Check in and move slower closer to the knee.

3. The short head of the biceps femoris takes a slight 45° angle medially to make contact.

4. Movements to ask for:

   - Lift foot up to ceiling
   - Press knee into table
   - Dorsiflex and plantar flex foot
   - Lift and tuck tailbone
   - Take tailbone to ceiling

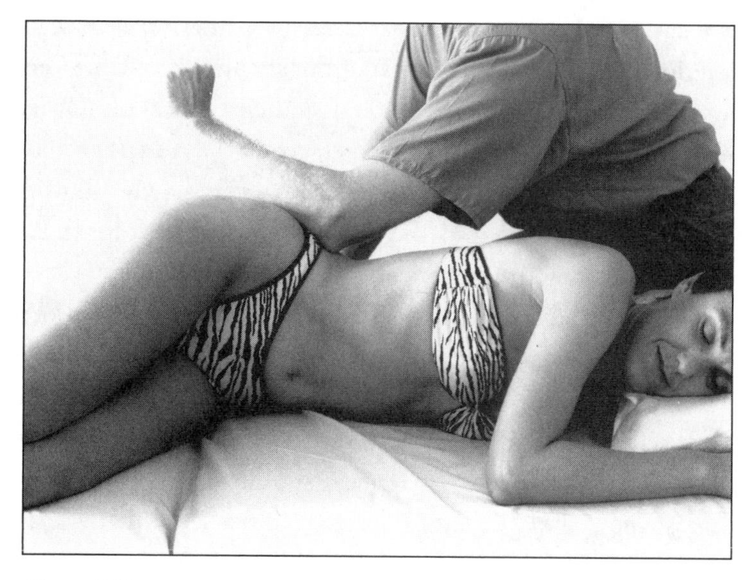

Figure 9.12

Postural Fascia over the Crest of the Ilium and the Greater Trochanter

The following are very basic techniques for releasing the superficial postural fascia of the lower leg and back. The client is in side lying position. You can see in Figure 9.12 that the therapist's body is placed behind the client and that the therapist is placing the elbow up against the crest of the ilium. The exact placement of his elbow is directly on the coronal plane of the body. To start this technique, place your elbow down into the waistline of the client before you make contact with the bone. Once you have gotten into the waistline, you can move your elbow up against the crest of the ilium. The contact is bone on bone. Incrementally build pressure of up to several pounds against the crest and hold that until you feel a softening or a spreading of the fascia over the hip. This is a very important area to work because eight major structures of the body cross the crest within several inches of the elbow. They are the quadratus lumborum, the peritonium, the gluteus maximus, the tensor fasciae latae, all three layers of the thoracal lumbar fascia, (the anterior, medial, and posterior), as well as all the fascia of the abdominal obliques, and the transversus and rectus abdominus muscles. If you do not feel softening occur with your gradual pressure on the crest, then allow your elbow to glide back toward the sacrum, very slowly following the bony ridge of the crest. The best movement to ask for in this position is tucking the tailbone forward and back.

Another good movement is to have the client flex her knee forward several inches and then back. The releases of the fascia on the bone can be quite different than normal muscle softening or relaxation. Sometimes it requires more concentration on the part of the therapist and it may happen more slowly than soft tissue releases. The technique here is different in the sense that you are maintaining a static stretch on a bony area of the body, holding it for several seconds, up to a minute, and concentrating on sensing a release. You very often will feel a release occur when the client takes a deep breath, or when you begin to feel the breath move into the tissue around where you are working.

Figure 9.13 shows a stretch of the abductor of the leg. The abductors of the leg act as a shock absorber for the legs in walking, running, and exercise in general. Consequently, they are wound tightly and are a major contributor to low back pain. The greater trochanter is an important landmark to work because of all the attachments that come into it. Begin by placing the tip of your elbow on the greater trochanter of the femur. Then make very slow, small circles around the trochanter, moving the entire circumference of the trochanter so you can feel where the gluteal muscles attach and if they are tight. You can feel where the rotators come in and attach to the trochanter. While you are working on the trochanter, ask the client to flex her knee very slightly, to extend her heel very slightly, or to tuck her tailbone back and forth. Really hunt for tight tissue around the trochanter and spend a lot of time here. When you find tight tissue, ask the client to medially and laterally rotate her hip with a flexed knee while pinning the tissue. Then glide off of the trochanter with your elbow, going right down the middle of the IT band several inches at a time. It is important to take a break every minute or so and allow the client to take several breaths before beginning again. Pace your work and do smaller increments as you get close to the knee.

> This work is not only beneficial for low back clients, but is particularly beneficial for any clients with knee problems, and especially for anyone who has had knee replacement surgery.

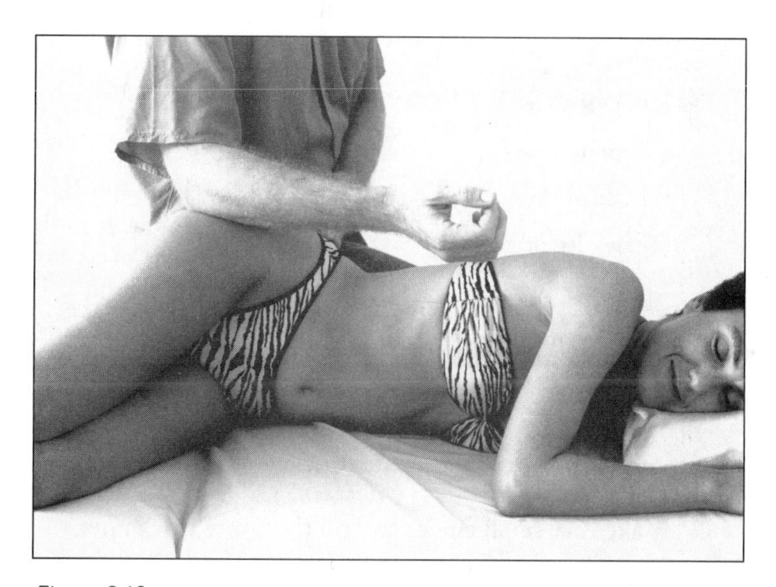

Figure 9.13

The Work: Postural Fascia over the Crest of the Ilium

Client Position: Side lying, with knees flexed at 45°

1. Place elbow up against the crest of the ilium directly on the coronal plane of the body.

2. Sink elbow down into the waistline before making contact with the bone.

3. Once connected, the direction of force will be inferior into the crest of the ilium.

4. Maintain steady pressure until a softening is felt.

5. If a softening is not felt, move posteriorly toward the sacrum following the iliac crest.

6. Movements to ask for:

   - Tuck the tailbone back and forth
   - Breath
   - Lengthen leg
   - Arm over head
   - Knee to chest
   - Bring leg off table

The Work: Greater Trochanter / IT Band

Client Position: Side lying, with knees flexed at 45°

1. Land gently onto the greater trochanter with the elbow.

2. Make very small circles around the entire trochanter.

3. Following tight tissues will take you into the IT band.

4. Make slow movements toward the knee searching for tight tissues.

5. Movements to ask for are:

   - Flex of the knee
   - Extend the hip and press through the heel

- Tuck tailbone back and forth
- "Rub a penny" between the knees
- Medially and laterally rotate hip

> You are moving over vastus lateralis when working in the IT band. Many trigger points can be found here too.

Gluteus Medius and the Tensor Fasciae Latae

The gluteus medius has a fascial compartment that goes the whole length of the lower leg. You can see in Figure 9.14 that the therapist is approaching the client from behind, and he is using the point of his elbow to sink very slowly into the area of the gluteus medius. This can be found by putting your finger on the crest of the ilium at the coronal plane. Just line up your finger on the coronal plane and then move your finger halfway down the line of the coronal plane toward the trochanter. Then place your elbow in that halfway point and very slowly give a direct medial compression into the hip until you make contact with the tight or restricted area. Once you have found the tight area of the gluteus medius, or the client has told you that it is sensitive, hold that area and very slowly have the client straighten her leg, stretch her heel, and move her leg back behind the coronal plane of the body, so that her lumbars arch anteriorly. Repeat this procedure several times and also have the client slowly flex her knee into her chest in order to get a full range of motion, not only in the hip joint, but also in the lower lumbars. There is also another direction of force that you are applying into the hip at this time. It is to move the hip and leg inferiorly. Once you have found the tight area with your medial compression, add the second vector of pressure into the leg by pushing the hip down toward the feet. Another vector to explore is to turn around and face the client's head. Enter as before on the coronal line, but vector up and under gluteus maximus and diagonally toward the iliac crest. The client will be more than happy to lead you to the best spot.

The tensor fasciae latae attaches to the anterior superior iliac spine (ASIS) and the greater trochanter. Friction or static pressure feels good on this muscle.

> This type of work can be very strong and should not be used on the acute low back client.

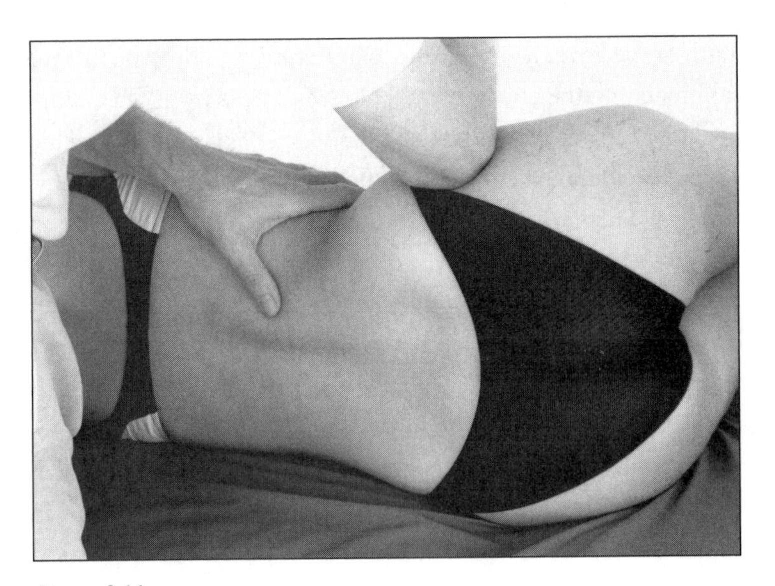

Figure 9.14

The Work: Gluteus Medius

Client Position: Side lying, with knees flexed at 45°

1. Standing behind the client, use the elbow point to gently sink into the area of the gluteus medius on the coronal plane.

2. Use medial compressional force until contacting the tight tissue.

3. If you turn around and face the client's head, there is a sweet or sensitive spot that is commonly found when the vector is medial and toward the iliac crest, as if attempting to get under the gluteus maximus.

4. To enhance the release, add a second vector by pushing the hip down toward the client's feet.

5. Movements to ask for:

- Extend hip
- Press through heel
- Move the leg back off the table
- Flex the knee to the chest

The Work: Tensor Fasciae Latae

Client Position: Side lying, with knees flexed at 45°

1. The tensor fasciae latae (TFL) attaches to the ASIS and the greater trochanter.

2. Once you have connected these two landmarks you are right in the TFL muscle.

3. Use deep sustained pressure to soften tissues or friction when necessary.

Quadriceps

For this technique, your point of contact should be very broad. Notice in Figure 9.15 that the therapist is using about 5 to 6 inches of his elbow over the quadriceps. Apply up to several pounds of compression into the quadriceps and ask the client to flex her knee an inch or two. The movement of the knee should also be done very slowly. This technique goes inferiorly from the top of the quadriceps, starting several inches inferior to the inguinal ligament. Cover several inches of territory on the leg and then stop, giving the client a break before going further. Some clients have tight quads closer to the inguinal ligaments, and some clients have tight quads down closer to her knee. Wherever they are most tight is where you can spend the most time making a gliding motion down toward the knee, or keeping your elbow in place and frictioning back and forth an inch or two at a time.

> This technique is also the beginning of the iliopsoas release. The psoas initiates movement in knee flexion. Although this movement is very slight, it is often overwhelmed by overactive quadriceps, which contributes to a lack of tone in the psoas.

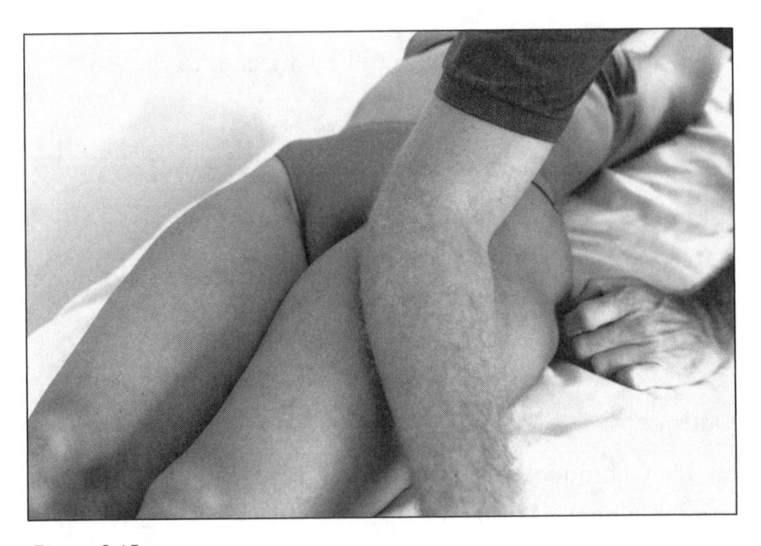

Figure 9.15

The Work: Quadriceps

Client Position: Supine

1. Using a broad elbow and several pounds of pressure, sink into the quadriceps muscle.

2. Move slowly from the top of the quadriceps to the knee.

3. Ask for flexion of the knee.

Septum between the Quadriceps and Adductors

In Figure 9.16 the therapist's hands are the septum between the quadriceps and the adductors. You start by applying pressure into the septum posteriorly and then move downward toward the knee. The best movement to ask for is to flex the knee back and forth. This release for the adductors is beneficial for your low back clients. The pressure you are applying in the septum is deep and sustained. This will also reflex into the floor of the pelvis and prevertebral fascia. If the client has the capacity, ask her to lift her tailbone up to the ceiling and alternately push her tailbone into the table while stretching the fascia. You can also coordinate dorsiflexion and plantar flexion of the foot and flexion of the knee as one movement. Gradually as the client becomes accustomed to this style of work, she will be able to accomplish more than one movement at a time.

> The treatment sequence is to work the adductors, then the psoas, and then the quadratus lumborum.

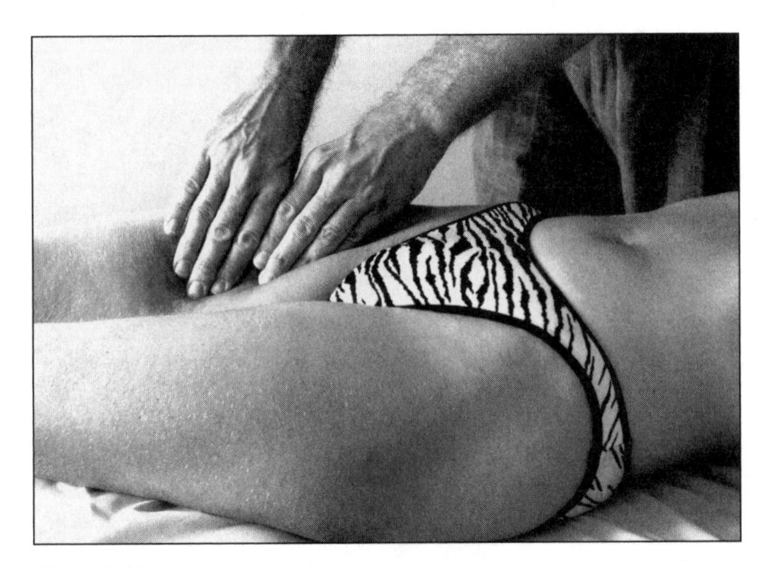

Figure 9.16

The Work: Septum between Quadriceps and Adductors

Client Position: Supine

1. Apply posterior pressure, deep and sustained, into the septum and move inferiorly toward the knee with hands or elbow.

2. Ask client to flex the knee back and forth or tilt pelvis very slowly.

3. Be mindful as there is a femoral artery near this area.

Be mindful of the Hunter's canal as you traverse inferiorly toward the knee. The Hunter's canal is a fascial sheath that surrounds a neurovascular bundle and can be extremely tender to the touch.

CHAPTER 10

Releases for the Shoulder and Arm

Clavicle, Coracoid Process, and Sternum

The client should be in supine position. Figure 10.1 shows the therapist palpating either end of the clavicle. Place your thumb or pisiform bone surface of both hands on the opposite ends of the individual clavicle and compress inferiorly and medially. Repeat slowly in unison with the breath until you feel the clavicle soften and release.

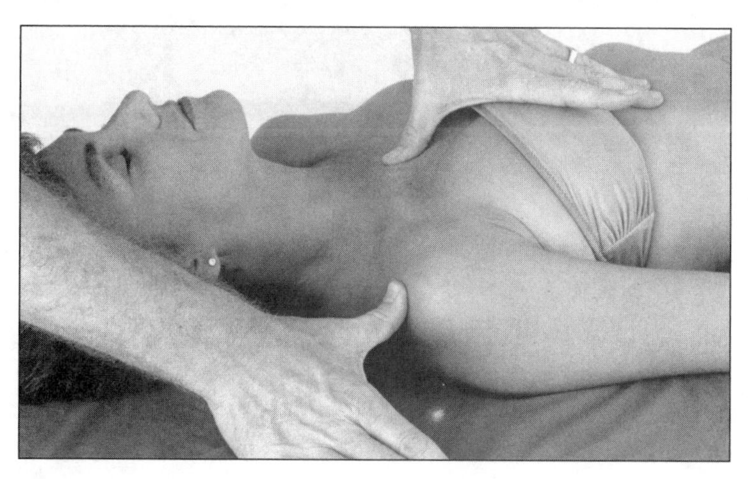

Figure 10.1

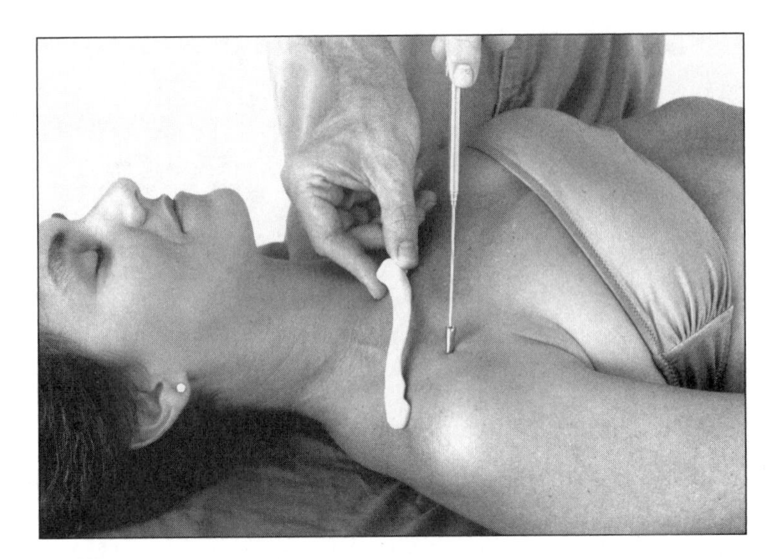

Figure 10.2

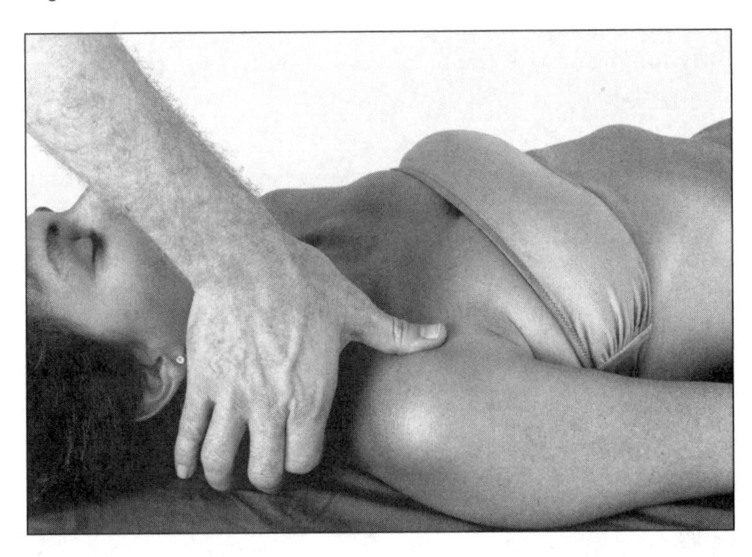

Figure 10.3

Next, palpate the coracoid process. Refer to Figure 10.2. Use the pisiform surface of your hand or thumb to compress posteriorly until its range of motion has increased. If it does not release, use your opposite hand to distract the distal end of the clavicle or alternate compression of each (coracoid process and clavicle) until a release occurs as in Figure 10.3.

To work the sternum, place the heel of your hand over the xiphoid process but not directly on it. Place the heel of your opposite hand over the sternum above the angle of Louis. The angle of Louis is the junction between the body and the manubrium of the sternum. Slowly compress both hands posteriorly and together. The release is obtained when the bone feels more resilient and has increased mobility.

The Work: Clavicle, Coracoid Process, and Sternum

Client Position: Supine

1. Palpate each end of clavicle by pressing inferiorly and medial.

2. Do this in unison with the breath until a release is felt.

3. Palpate coracoid process posteriorly until the range of motion increases.

4. Place the heel of hand over xiphoid and the heel of opposite hand over the angle of Louis and press posteriorly until the range of motion increases.

Subclavian Muscle

The release of the subclavian muscle is a favorite technique. The therapist has placed a clavicle on the client in Figure 10.4, pointing to where the subclavian muscle is in relation to the rest of the skeleton. As you can see in Figure 10.5, the client is in side lying position while the therapist's thumb is forming a wedge in between the clavicle and first rib, and his opposite hand is holding the shoulder around the deltoid. The key to this technique is to elevate the shoulder you are working on up toward the ear, thus elevating the clavicle. This

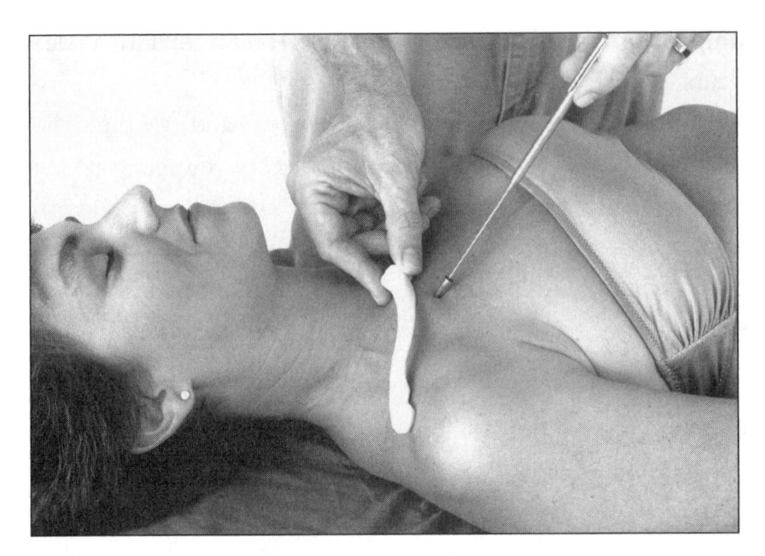

Figure 10.4

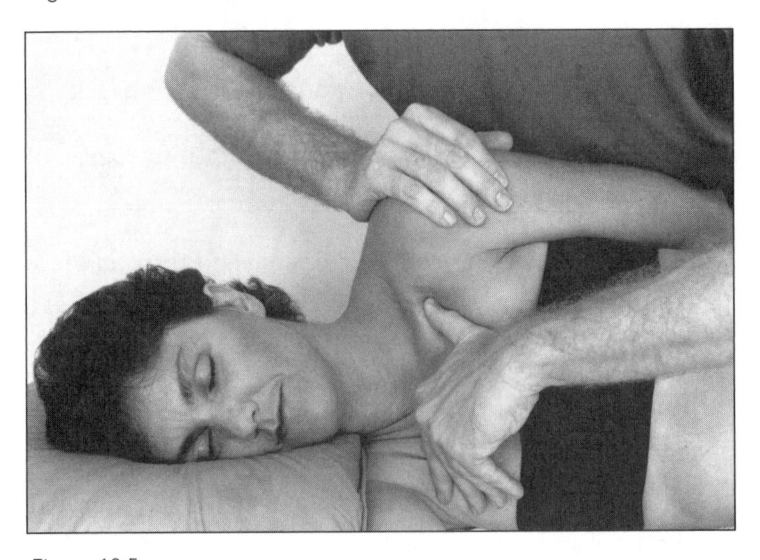

Figure 10.5

will allow you much deeper access into the subclavian muscle. Start your pressure right at the sternum between the clavicle and first rib. Move the shoulder up and attempt to hook your thumb under the clavicle as though you were going to stretch the periosteum of the

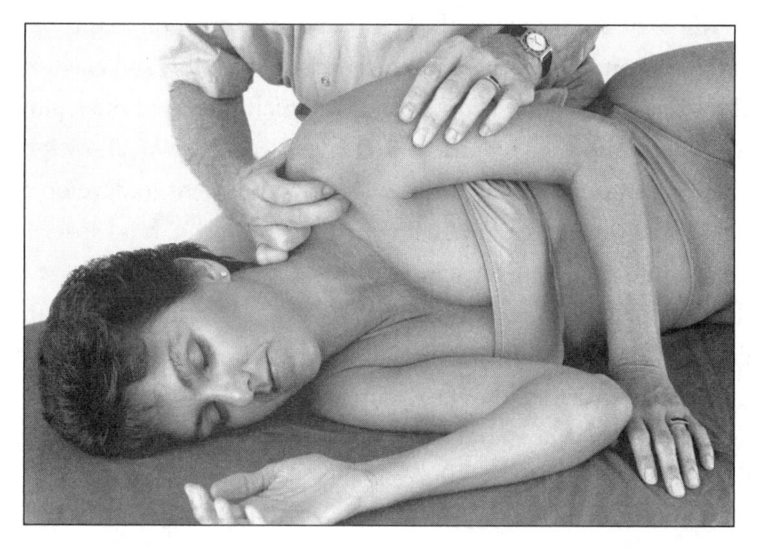

Figure 10.6

clavicle. Move a half an inch at a time along the underside of the clavicle, and in the first several inches, you will feel what appears to be a tight band, which is the subclavian muscle. As you apply pressure, which in this case can be 5 to 10 pounds, you will feel that ligament begin to soften. But do not stop there. Continue your search under the clavicle, moving distally very slowly until you reach the coracoid process.

This is a good stretch for the clavipectoral fascia, and as you get closer to the coracoid process, you will run into the conoid and trapezoid ligaments that attach the clavicle to the coracoid process. With your thumb or your fingers, as shown in Figure 10.6, forming a wedge in between the coracoid process and the clavicle, maintain a static pressure until you feel those ligaments start to stretch. Do not forget to use the opposite hand to elevate and slightly circumduct the shoulder while doing this. It is as though you are using the clavicle as a stick shift and you are attempting to find the right gear that will allow the release. There is some coordination needed between your right hand and your left hand.

Make sure you observe the before and after position of the clavicle. With any technique around the trunk, the ribs, and clavicles, always ask the client at the end of the technique to take a slow, full breath into the area that was just worked. This will allow for a much greater release and again will allow the client to develop an internal awareness of any changes that have gone on. It is especially important because of the connection the lungs and pleura have to the first rib. The subclavian artery is in between the clavicle and first rib. Whenever the subclavian muscle is tight, it will obstruct the subclavian artery. The vertebral artery branches off the right and left subclavian arteries and weaves its way up into the head through the transverse processes of the cervical vertebra. The vertebral artery then branches off to form three other arteries: the basilar, cerebella, and meningeal arteries. If you suspect cerebral vascular insufficiency is present in a client, it will be well worth your effort to free the subclavian muscle.

The Work: Subclavian Muscle

Client Position: Side lying, with knees flexed 45°

1. Using thumb, form a wedge in between the inferior aspect of the clavicle and first rib at the sternum.

2. With the other hand, elevate the shoulder upward toward the ear.

3. Search for tight bands moving medial from the sternum toward the coracoid process.

4. Do not forget to use the opposite hand to elevate or circumduct the shoulder while doing this.

5. Cue the client to take slow, deep breaths into the area that was just worked.

Superficial Fascia of the Arm

The fascia of the arms is continuous with the cervical fascia and is often overlooked. As seen in Figure 10.7, you may have the client lay prone, and her head can be turned in either direction. You can experiment with the head position by turning it to the opposite direction and seeing if that shortens the arm that you are working on and vice versa. Take your fingertips right over the attachment of the deltoid muscle in the upper arm and get hold of as much of the superficial fascia of the arm as you can. While you are moving down the arm inferiorly, several inches at a time, you can have the client lift her head and slowly turn it one way and then the other. Alternately you will also have her bend her elbow slowly toward the side of her body and back as well as dorsiflexing the wrist and hand.

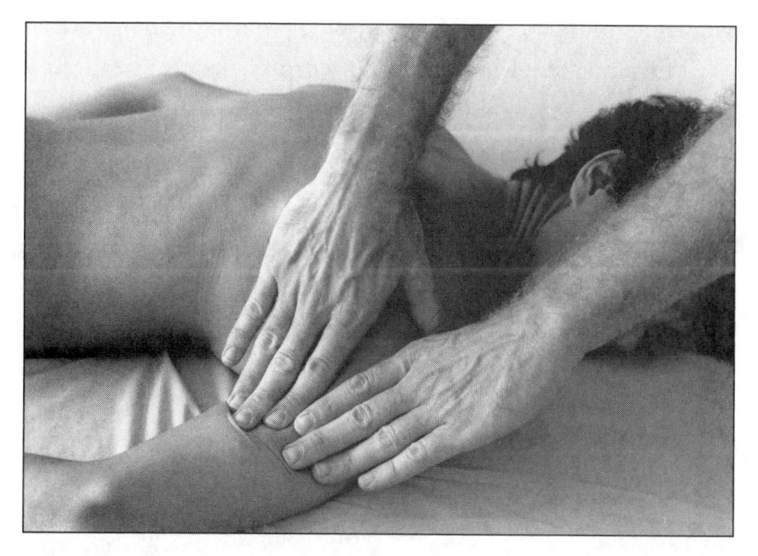

Figure 10.7

What is really liked about this technique is that you can go down the entire length of the arm. While around the elbow, it is convenient to work the fascia off of the olecranon process. Below the elbow, you can get much more deeply into the interosseous membrane of the forearm. While working deeply in the forearm in this manner, have the client roll her arm very slightly back and forth or pronate then supinate the forearm, but very slowly so it does not throw your fingers out of position. Although Figure 10.8 does not show it here, you can certainly keep going right down over the retinaculum of the wrist and work that tissue in the same way as you did the retinaculum over the ankle. It is here that you would be more active with wrist flexion while you are working that fascia. This technique is found to be particularly beneficial for anyone that has had a whiplash injury, and they were the driver of the car. Also, the numerous ways in which back problems occur from lifting can also be treated very nicely this way. Remember that the fascia of the arm goes in four basic directions when they meet at the shoulder girdle: to the TMJ, to the scalenes, to the upper trunk muscles, and to the lower trunk muscles. You will really enjoy this particular work as a way of finishing any work done on the trunk, neck, or head. As an alternative, you can have the client turn her head slowly while you are working the arm. This will assist the cervical fascia to release.

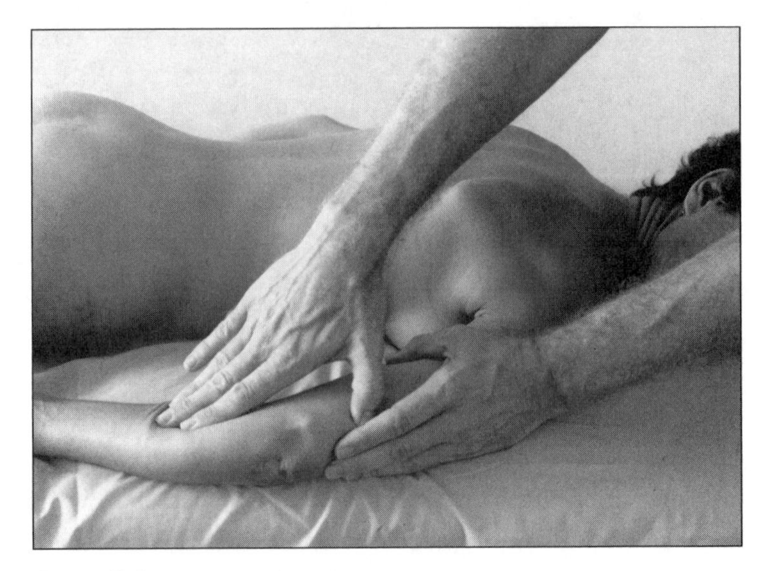

Figure 10.8

These techniques are effective for local problems in the arm or as a way to finish up neck work.

The Work: Superficial Fascia of the Arm

Client Position: Prone

1. Fingertips begin in the posterior deltoid muscle moving superficial fascia down the arm inferiorly several inches at a time.

2. The vector is in and down the arm.

3. Client lifts her head, slowly turning one way or another, as well as dorsiflexing the wrist and hand.

4. While around the elbow, work the olecranon process and deeply into the interosseous membrane of the forearm.

5. Have the client roll her arm back and forth slightly.

6. Using an elbow while working the forearm, if necessary.

Clavipectoral and Deltoid Fasciae

In some respects, these techniques are the same as those of the superficial fascia of the arm. However, these flexors of the arm tend to be the most problematic. You may start with your fingertips or elbow right at the head of the humerus, very close to the coracoid process as shown in Figure 10.9. The deltoid is stretched while the client has her palm down on the table and periodically moves her elbow toward the side of her body and back out. Tell the client to imagine she has a dime under her elbow, and she is trying to slide

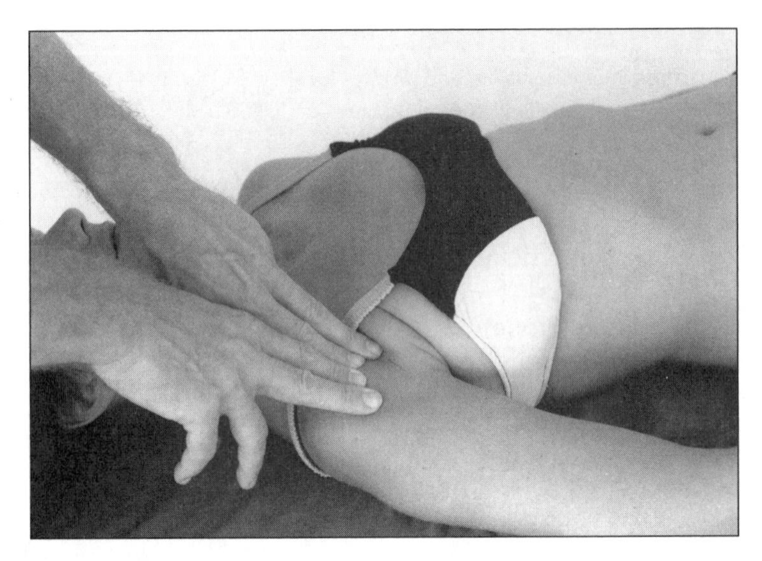

Figure 10.9

that dime toward her body and back out. This way, she does not have the temptation to lift her elbow and rotate it in order to move it toward her body. This type of movement gives greater access to the deeper fasciae of the arm and thus the entire body. As before, only move several inches at a time and then give the client a break and occasionally ask her to take a breath into the area you just worked.

Spend time around the anterior deltoid as well as the middle deltoid because this is where the fascia will usually bunch up. The direction of movement is from the top of the shoulder down toward the elbow, and you can spend several minutes on each deltoid. You can even clean some of the tissue off of the distal end of the clavicle, as well as over the coracoid process, if it is buried with a lot of tissue that has resulted from injuries to the upper girdle. The important thing with this technique is to keep the arm and hand as flat as possible on the table. This requires the client to keep some degree of tension in her arm to maintain this position. The tendency is for the arm to pop up when pressure is applied over the head of the humerus. You can use your opposite hand to hold down the wrist if

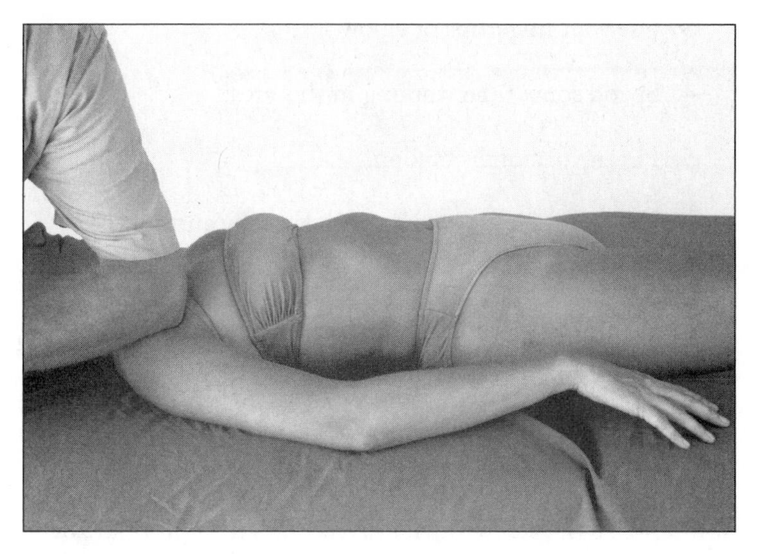

Figure 10.10

you need to. When you ask the client to move her elbow in and out, have her make small movements. She does not need to move any more than an inch or two at a time. The movement should be done slowly to affect the deeper fasciae and the interosseous membrane. You can work down into the biceps or laterally over the edge of the humerus. Another option is to pin the pectoralis tendon in the glenohumeral joint, as shown in Figure 10.10, and have the client rotate her shoulder laterally and then stretch her arm down to her foot. Wait for a softening and then return to neutral and disengage.

The Work: Clavipectoral and Deltoid Fascia

Client Position: Supine

1. Fingertips begin in the deltoid muscle moving superficial fascia down the arm inferiorly several inches at a time.

2. Client can imagine she has a dime under her elbow and is trying to move it toward her body and back out.

3. Use your fingertips or elbow.

4. Spend some time working in this area.

5. Pin the pectoralis tendon.

6. Have the client rotate her arm laterally and stretch it down toward her feet.

7. Wait for a softening and return to neutral.

Teres Major and Minor

Place your elbow just slightly inferior to the axillary border and just inferior to the acromion. Pause and sink to appropriate depth. Your vector or line of drive is on the coronal plane toward the midline. Instruct the client that when you happen upon a tender spot or a tight spot that you will pause, they can slowly internally and externally rotate their shoulder (Figure 10.11). This is like a pin and stretch, and is very effective in treating those attachments. Glide slowly along the axillary border, and once you have reached the inferior angle lighten your pressure and come off. You can repeat this three or four times, or as the client can tolerate. This release can be used for any shoulder problems.

The Work: Teres Major and Minor

Client Position; Prone, with arm hanging off the table at a 90° angle

1. Face the feet and place elbow on the coronal line of the axillary border just inferior to the spine of the scapula.

2. Search for tight tissue.

3. Movement to ask for:

   - Internally and externally rotate shoulder

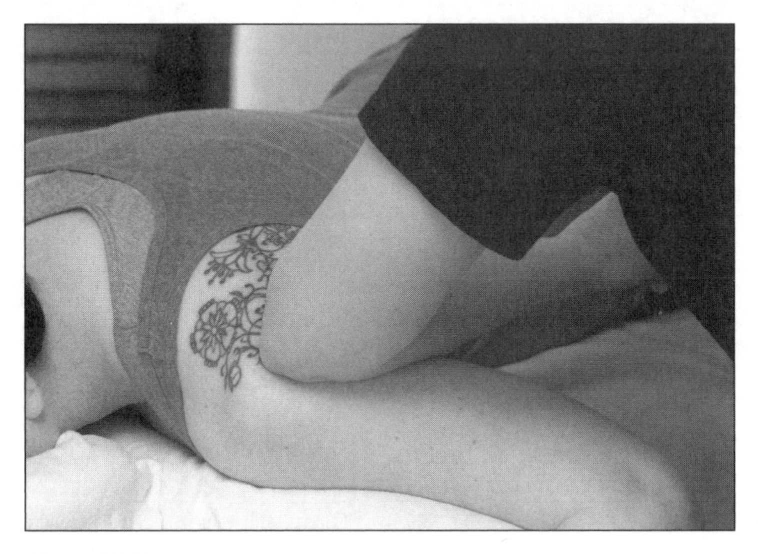

Figure 10.11

Subscapularis Muscles and Pectoralis Minor

Begin the work on the subscapularis by approaching the axilla directly on the coronal plane of the body with the client in supine position and her arm at a 90° angle. Palpate with the pads of your fingertips against the rib as shown in Figure 10.12. Press into the ribs to mobilize them, and at the same time, follow the ribs around posteriorly at an angle toward T4. When your fingers cannot go any further, you have bumped right up against the subscapularis. At this point, ask the client to extend her arm over her head very slowly while you hold the subscapularis. Remember to have her take a breath when she brings her arm down. Another option is to have her take her arm up to the ceiling, and horizontally adduct her arm to her chest. This puts her scapula in to your fingertips.

To release pectoralis minor, all you do is turn your hand around and enter into the axilla at the coronal plane, as before, and slide your fingers over the ribs toward the manubriumas shown in Figure 10.13.When your fingers cannot go any further, you have contacted

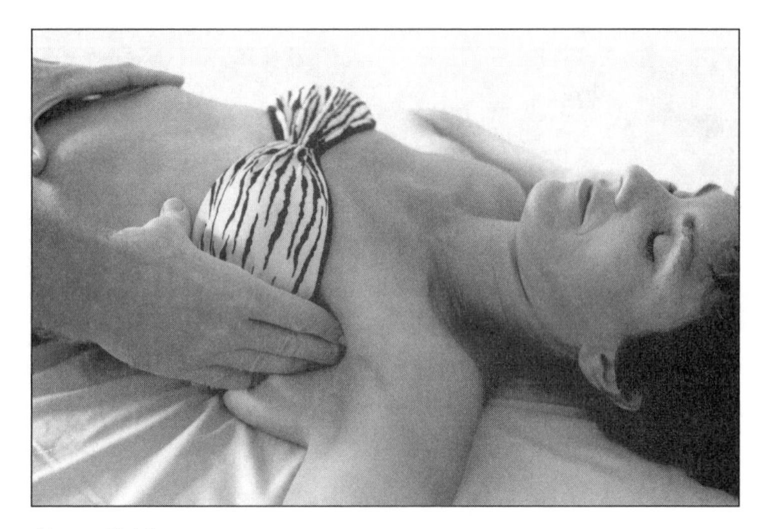

Figure 10.12

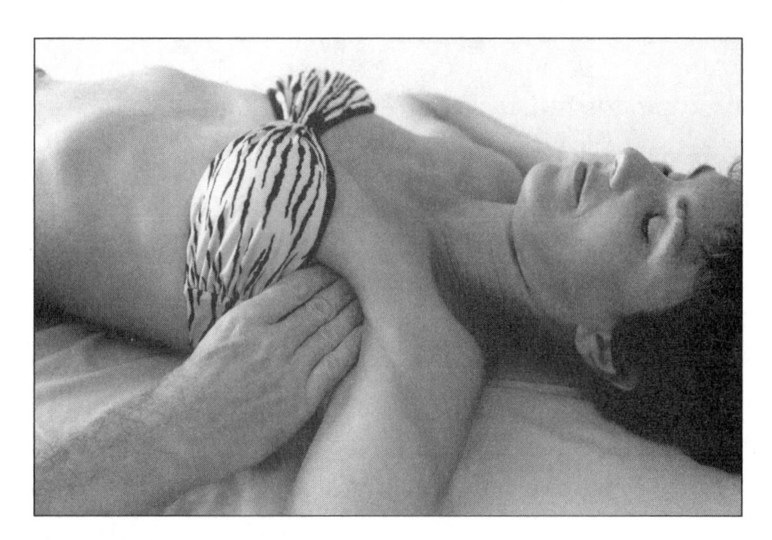

Figure 10.13

the pectoralis minor. Then repeat the same procedure as before: ask the client to extend her arms slowly over her head and occasionally have her take a breath into the point of contact. It is not unusual for the client to report a burning sensation, which is indicative of the fascia stretching. You should not usually repeat the axilla work more than two or three times. Remember that this is a very sensitive area, so go slowly, yet firmly.

> The brachial plexus is sometimes entrapped by the pectoralis minor causing numbness, tingling, and weakness down the arm. Make sure a medical professional has ruled out any pathologies of the thoracic or cervical spine. This technique is very effective for anyone who has a shortening of the pectoralis minor from trauma, poor posture, or repetitive motion injuries.

Many students start too low and end up stretching the serratus anterior. Aim your hand directly into the axilla at the mid coronal plane of the body. Keep the pads of your fingers up against the ribs. Always motion test the ribs you are on before you proceed. Press into the ribs very slowly with several pounds of pressure. If they feel hard and resistant to the pressure, then they are stuck. Maintain a firm pressure on them and ask the client to breathe into your point of contact. Within two or three cycles of respiration, you should feel the rib start to move. Then continue moving the tips of your fingers around in the direction described above. If the client reports sensitivity, ask her to breathe into the point of contact. Repeat this procedure several times. Each time see if the client can reach even higher over her head. As she returns her arm down to the starting position, have her inhale again as you lighten up your contact.

This work is very effective for neck and shoulder problems because it opens up the clavipectoral fasciae and deep cervical fasciae.

The Work: Subscapularis

Client Position: Supine, with arm at 45°

1. Approach the axilla on the coronal plane and gently make contact with the ribs.
2. Mobilize the ribs to check for movement.
3. Angle fingers down and slightly inferiorly toward T4, feeling for the border of subscapularis.
4. Ask the client to extend her arm over her head.
5. Another option is to horizontally adduct the client's arm, and the scapula will begin to abduct.
6. This will make it easier to come into contact with the anterior surface of the scapula.
7. Ask for a breath and wait for a softening.
8. Friction can be used when indicated.
9. Ask for breath when coming out of the release.

The Work: Pectoralis Minor

Client Position: Supine, with arm at 45°

1. Approach the axilla on the coronal plane and gently make contact with the ribs.

2. Mobilize the ribs to assess for movement.

3. Angle fingers up and over toward the manubrium.

4. When fingers cannot go any further, you are in contact with pectoralis minor.

5. Ask the client to extend her arm slowly over her head.

6. Occasionally ask for breath into the area of contact.

7. May repeat two to three times.

8. This is a very sensitive area. Enter mindfully.

Biceps and Extensor Compartment of the Forearm

Figure 10.14 shows the therapist using a broad, soft fist to stretch the bicep. Your ability to move from a broad surface to a smaller surface depends on the tool you are using. Fingertips or knuckles allow you to do some detail work on individual spots of the fascial bag that are stuck. With a slight switch in the position of your hand

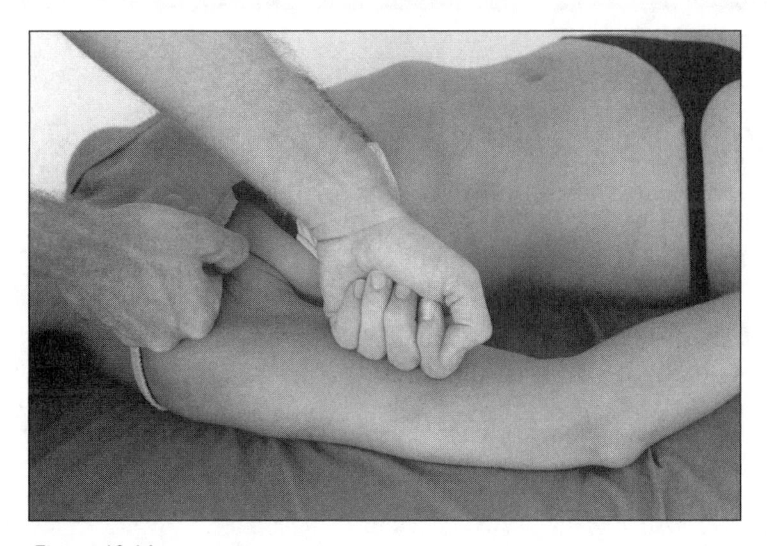

Figure 10.14

to fist or elbow, you can take that release into a much broader plane of fascia. This is called organizing the fascia. As with the preceding techniques, keep the arm and hand as flat as possible on the table so the technique can be more effective and use the same type of elbow movement as before. Now it will be a little more challenging for the client to flex her elbow in and out since you are applying more pressure close to the elbow.

Once you get below the elbow, you like to get the point of your own elbow on top of the extensor compartment and very slowly move straight down several inches at a time toward the wrist. Figure 10.15 shows the therapist pointing with his finger where your elbow is to be placed. This is a very strong action because the motion you are asking the client to make is extending the wrist up, and in this case, ask the client to focus on pointing her fingertips toward the ceiling. Remember do not hold that as a static stretch, but to ask her to relax her hand occasionally. The closer you get with your elbow to the wrist, you need to think about whether or not you are going to switch tools and use your fingertips and knuckles to go over the retinaculum and carpal bones. In some cases with large wrists, you can continue right on over the wrist with your elbow and you need not be afraid to use

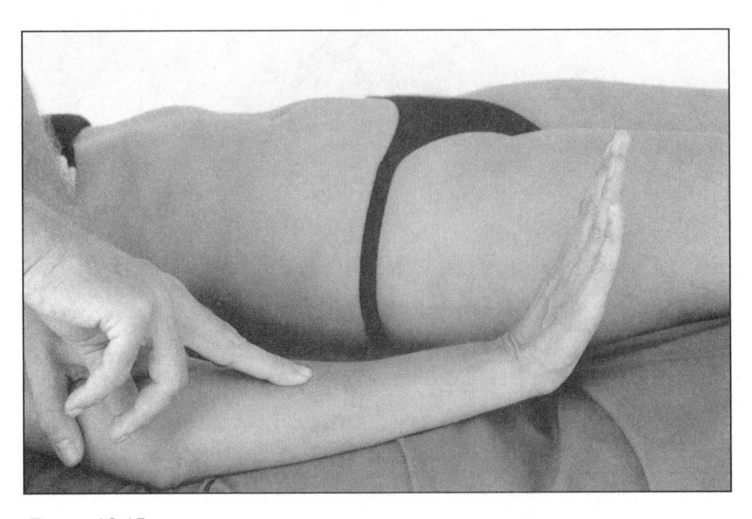

Figure 10.15

a lot of pressure. This work is particularly beneficial for any driver in an automobile accident and the increasing number of repetitive motion injuries that occur in the wrist and the elbow, especially computer work station folks and the like.

The Work: Biceps and Extensor Compartment of the Forearm

Client Position: Supine

1. Use fist from deltoid to elbow, moving from a broad surface to a smaller surface when necessary.

2. Once below the client's elbow, use the elbow point on top of the extensor compartment.

3. Moving inferiorly down several inches at a time while asking the client to flex and extend her wrist.

Extensor Retinaculum of the Wrist and the Flexor Compartment of the Forearm

These techniques are especially beneficial to those clients that have had repetitive motion injuries to the wrist and forearms. In Figure 10.16,the therapist is pressing down directly on top of the carpal bone with the flat portion of his knuckle. Another option is to use six fingers. The client has her hand lying flat on the table. The elbow is also flat on the table and pronated. The therapist begins over the retinaculum of the wrist slightly superior to where Figure 10.16 shows, then he gradually works his way down into the wrist and hands. Start on the midline of the forearm or actually in between the radius and the ulna. This is very similar to the work on the ankle in that you start on the midline, get contact with the tissue over the bone by touching into the bone, and then add a second vector by spreading the tissue laterally away from the midline. As you spread

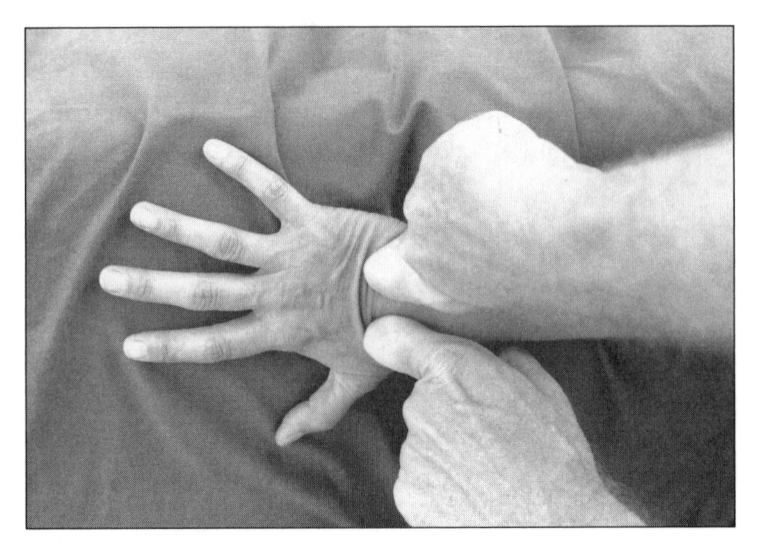

Figure 10.16

the tissue down into the wrist and away from the midline, you can also ask the client to bend her elbow in toward her body slowly and then back out. This will have a very big effect on the interosseous membrane, as well as the carpal tunnel. This is another area of the body where the superficial fasciae and deep fasciae of the body merge at the surface or outer layer of the body. People with chronic upper girdle problems have rarely had work below the level of their elbow. You must remember, however, that all of these fasciae are interconnected, and most everyone has had numerous falls on their hands and wrists at some time in their life.

The interosseous membrane is an excellent entry point into work for the whole arm, shoulder girdle, neck, TMJ, and trunk.

In Figure 10.17, the therapist is working on the flexor compartments of the forearm and also the interosseous membrane. This is a

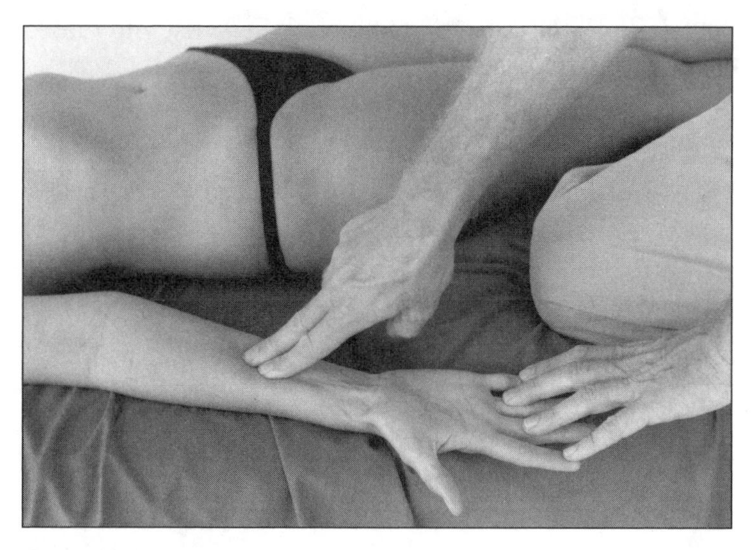

Figure 10.17

very effective and simple technique and begins right over the carpal tunnel of the wrist and continues all the way up to the elbow. The pressure is deep, firm, and continuous for several inches at a time. The client should be reminded to keep her fingers stretched and extended while you are working, and she can also roll her forearm by pronating and supinating occasionally while you are in between the radius and the ulna. When you get close to the elbow, you can then ask the client to flex her forearm slightly, and this will have an effect on the fascia of the coracobrachialis and biceps muscles. All in all, these two techniques are the ones that you may use consistently with clients with upper extremity problems, and especially for TMJ and cervical whiplash. Remember that the driver in every single whiplash case is usually gripping the steering wheel very powerfully, and the point of impact causes a force vector to come through the hands and wrists directly. Again, this is a forgotten element in the treatment of high velocity impact traumas.

The Work: Extensor Retinaculum of the Wrist and the Flexor Compartment of the Forearm

Client Position: Supine

1. To work extensor retinaculum, have client pronate her forearm with hand flat to table.

2. Start at the midline over the retinaculum of the wrist.

3. Apply pressure using flat knuckles or fingers and spread laterally working down into the wrist and hand.

4. Client can slowly bend elbow toward her body and back out in small movements.

5. To work flexor compartment, have client supinate her forearm with an open palm.

6. Start at the carpal tunnel of the wrist.

7. Apply pressure using fingers or elbow and work up to the elbow.

8. Keep pressure deep and continuous, and move only a few inches at a time.

9. Client can slowly pronate and supinate forearm while working between ulna and radius.

10. Client can flex her forearm while working close to the elbow.

CHAPTER 11

Releases of Neck, Head, and Face

Sternocleidomastoid and Superficial Cervical Fascia

This technique is an excellent way of organizing the superficial fascia of the neck. Be mindful that you are not applying pressure into the neck with this technique. Instead, you are using broad contact with a very soft fist. Begin directly on top of the sternocleidomastoid, SCM. From there, you glide off the SCM and work your way around to the spinous processes of the cervical vertebrae. The moment you begin gliding with your fist, have the client begin to turn her head slowly in the opposite direction. The best way for the cervical fascia to lengthen is with a twisting motion. You can repeat this procedure three or four times on each side, and the more comfortable you become with the technique, the more pressure you can use. The pressure on the neck is certainly not going to be as great as on other areas of the body because of the delicate structures located in the neck, particularly the carotid artery.

The Work: Sternocleidomastoid and Superficial Cervical Fascia

Client Position: Supine

1. Using broad, four finger contact, make a very relaxed fist and place it over the SCM.

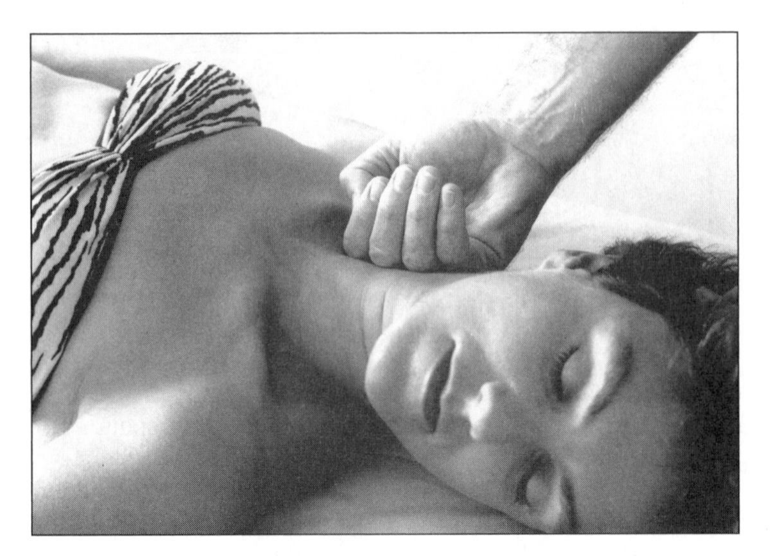

Figure 11.1

2. Do not apply a great deal of pressure, just make contact.

3. Move posteriorly around to the spinous processes of the cervical vertebrae as the client turns her neck in the opposite direction.

4. Repeat this procedure three to four times.

5. Be sure to enter the tissue and then immediately move off at an oblique angle.

Use soft seeing skills to avoid any defensive splinting that activates the sympathetic nervous system. Keep your vision softly trained on the client for breath changes, skin color changes, shaking, or tremoring, all of this being a sign of autonomic nervous system activation. Three sympathetic ganglia come together here. Work slowly and communicate frequently.

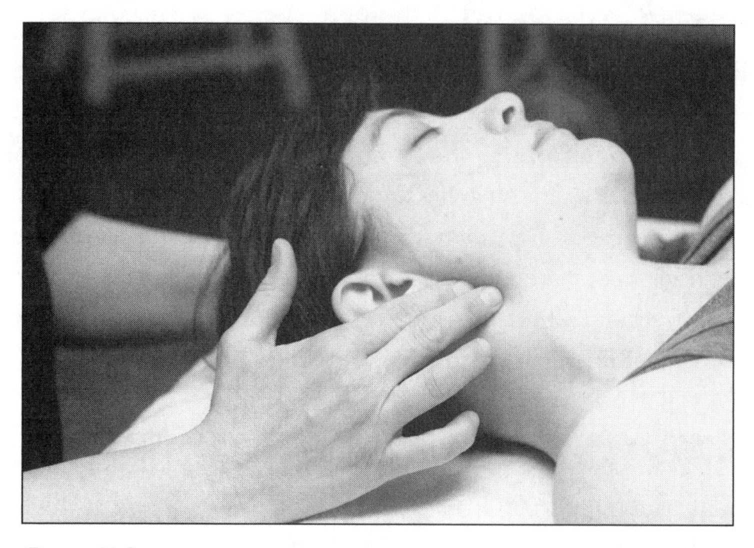

Figure 11.2

Digastric

The digastric is known for its two bellies. One belly attaches at the mastoid process deep to the SCM, and the second attaches to the inferior border of the mandible. Take a look in your anatomy book to get a good sense of this important, yet neglected muscle.

The client is supine and you are sitting at the head of the table. Cradle the head to one side. Place the thumb of your working hand on the mastoid process, as shown in Figure 11.2, and start to apply some appropriate pressure while searching for tight tissue. The attachment of digastric lives under the SCM on the anterior portion of the mastoid process. Begin to glide inferiorly a few inches and begin to soften this attachment. You usually glide through this area at least 10 times, working anteriorly to posteriorly from and around the mastoid process. Keep these glides short, as you have the carotid artery in your path. Of course, if you feel a pulse, redirect your vector or lighten and come off altogether. When you are on the posterior belly at the mastoid process, you are also in the area of the styloid process. This process is quite fragile, so be careful with your pressure behind the ear.

The second part is to start again sitting at the head of the table. Place the pads of your fingertips just under the chin on the anterior belly and glide superiorly following or tracing the mandible up to the hyoid bone as shown in Figure 11.3. Be mindful of the submandibular gland that lies under the mandible. A good amount of pressure can be used on both bellies of this muscle. You can treat any trigger points you find along the way. You can also ask the client to protract and retract the chin to emphasize this release. This work is excellent for clients with TMJ or forward head posture.

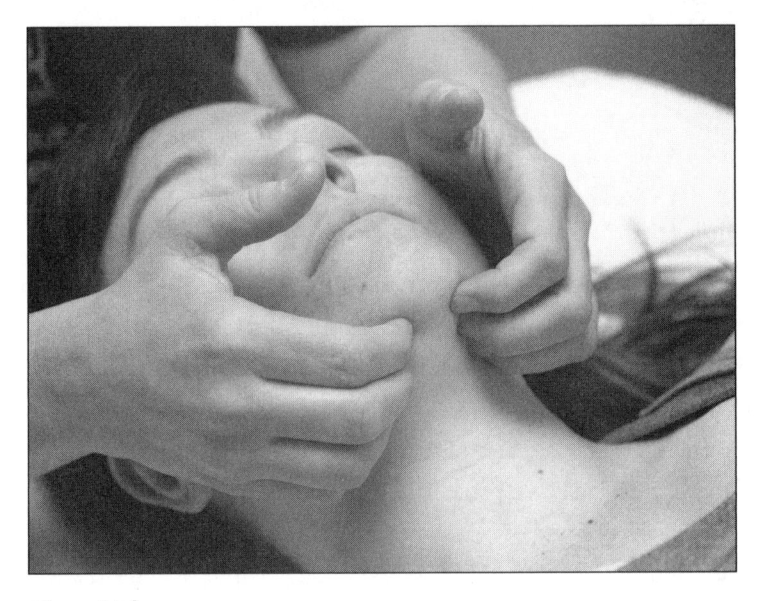

Figure 11.3

The Work: Digastric

Client Position: Supine

1. Place thumb on the mastoid process.

2. Use 10 to 12 short deep glides to soften the attachment of the digastric and the SCM.

3. Be mindful of the carotid artery.

4. Place fingertips under the chin at the digastric fossa.

5. With vector up toward the head, begin to trace the mandible superiorly ending at the hyoid bone. Repeat three to five times or as the client tolerates.

6. Be mindful of the submandibular gland.

7. Search and treat trigger points along the way.

8. Movements to ask for:

    - Protract and retract chin

Scalenes in Supine

The scalenes—anterior, middle, and posterior—come closest to the surface of the neck directly on the coronal plane midway between the occiput and the clavicle. Your fingers are directly posterior to the sternocleidomastoid muscle. Ask the client to lift her head slightly off the table, which activates the SCM. This makes it much easier to locate the scalenes. Begin by letting your fingers palpate the scalenes in their belly right where the therapist's fingers are located in Figure 11.4.Slightly side bend the neck toward the side you are working on and see if the tissue will soften indirectly. Then press more deeply into the scalenes incrementally and have the client slowly turn her head away from your hands. As she turns her head, you will also have the client tuck her chin up and down at the same time that she is turning her head. You will then begin gliding with your fingers intermittently down along the length of the scalenes until you get underneath the clavicle. Do this slowly and have her repeat the same turning and tucking motion with her head as before. This procedure can be repeated up to three times on each side of the neck.

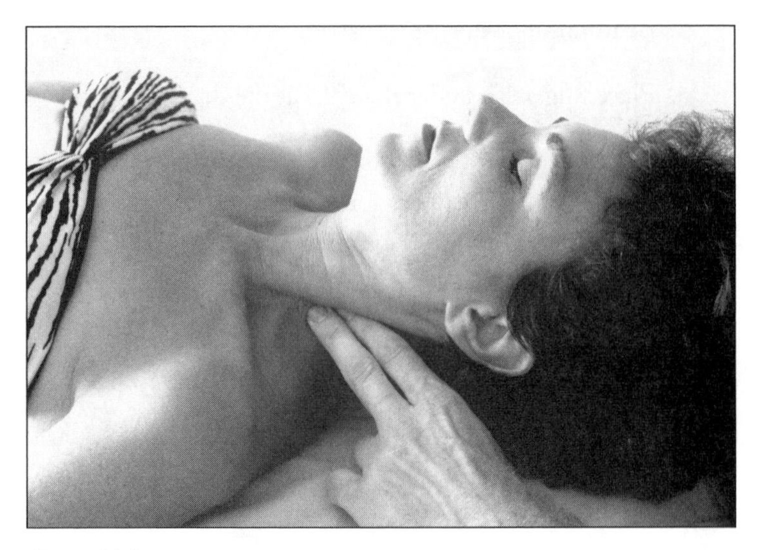

Figure 11.4

This area of the neck is very sensitive in those people with pathology and dysfunction in the cervicals. Because the scalenes assist in elevating the upper two ribs, you should always finish each technique by having the client take a deep breath into her upper rib cage, which will help facilitate an even greater opening for the work you are doing on the scalenes.

The Work: Scalenes

Client Position: Supine

1. Place fingers posterior to the SCM.

2. Ask client to lift her head to activate the SCM for better placement.

3. Once on the scalenes, side bend the neck into the side being worked to initiate a softening indirectly.

4. Adding a little deeper pressure, instruct the client to turn her head away from the side being worked.

5. The client can also tuck her chin up and down at the same time she is turning her head.

6. Glide fingers inferiorly down the length of the scalenes until the clavicle is reached.

7. Gently vector under the clavicle toward the ribs to work the attachments to the ribs.

8. Be mindful of the brachial plexus which runs in between middle and anterior scalene.

> The brachial plexus passes through the anterior and middle scalenes. While doing any anterior neck work, be very mindful of this endangerment site.

Scalenes, Trapezius, and Levator Scapula in Side Lying

These are some favorite techniques to use as a follow up to the supine scalene work. With the client in side lying, you can either support the head with a pillow or not depending on the amount of stretch you want to have. Using your free hand to stabilize the shoulder and arm, as shown in Figure 11.5, slightly distract it. Using several fingers of your working hand, begin at the lateral border of the trap and trace the border of the trapezius all the way up to occiput. During this journey from the lateral border of the trap to occiput, you will also have the occasion to run across the capitus levator and even the scalene muscles. This is an excellent stretch and mobilization of the fascia of the trunk and shoulder girdle and neck. It also feels wonderful to be on the receiving end of this. Remember that you

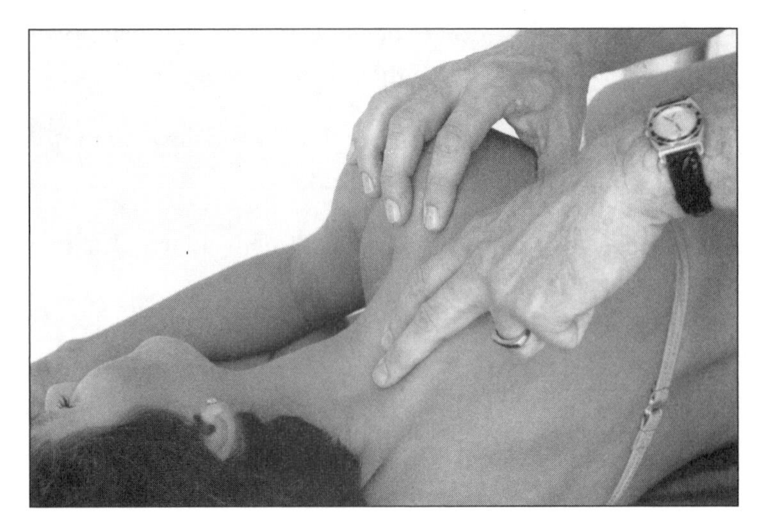

Figure 11.5

are keeping some dynamic tension by distracting the shoulder and arm with your free hand and moving the tissue of the neck in the opposite direction toward the head. You can repeat this procedure three to five times on each side.

Figure 11.5 shows the therapist with his fingers slightly anterior over the midline of the neck, which again places him either on top of the scalenes or the sternocleidomastoid. So in essence, you are working both the superficial and deep cervical fascia with this technique. Begin by palpating the trapezius and working that muscle and then the levator scapula. Then if you still want to spend time on the scalenes, go to it. You will find a flow with this technique by working back and forth from scalenes to traps back to scalenes to the sternocleidomastoid and so forth. The client can also assist by turning her head slightly, tucking her chin, or even lifting her head slightly off the table. Another way of having the client assist is by having her distract her arm and shoulder by placing her wrist over the head of her femur and asking her to reach for her toes. Whatever you can do to get her into the manipulation will be helpful.

The Work: Scalenes, Trapezius, and Levator Scapula

Client Position: Side lying, with knees flexed 45°

1. Stabilize the shoulder and slightly distract inferiorly with free hand.

2. Trace the border of the trapezius to the occiput with fingertips or knuckles of working hand.

3. Repeat three to five times.

4. Work back and forth from scalenes to trapezius to SCM to levator scapula; cover the entire area.

5. Movements to ask for:

    - Turn head slightly
    - Tuck chin
    - Move head off the table
    - Lift head slightly
    - Distract shoulder toward feet

Treatment for Cervical Whiplash

These are techniques used for treating chronic, but never acute, cervical whiplash problems. The base of the cervical spine ends at the level of T3, and this technique is a treatment for C7-T5. The client is in prone position with her head turned one way or the other. At the beginning, it does not make too much difference. You begin by placing the point of your elbow in the lamina groove just opposite or alongside the spinous process of the vertebrae starting at C7. Gradually apply pressure into the ribs and transverse processes and have her breathe into the point of contact to make sure you are not going too deep. Then slowly glide your elbow, maintaining pressure down several inches, while at the same time the client slowly lifts

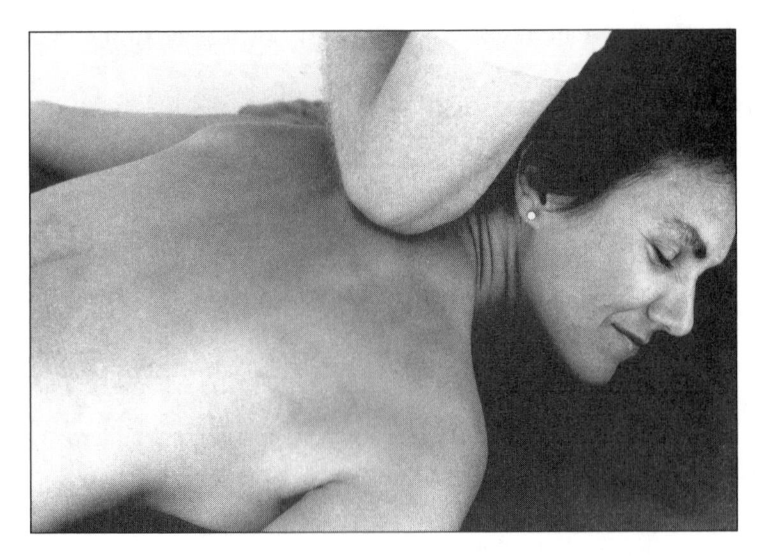

Figure 11.6

her head and turns it to the other side. The key here is to make sure that she pushes her breath into the point of contact while she is turning her head and while you are maintaining pressure as shown in Figure 11.6 and Figure 11.7. Repeat this procedure up to three times on each side and each lamina groove, starting with light pressure and finally building up to the heaviest pressure the client can tolerate. If she cannot breathe into the point of contact, then you cannot do the technique with the pressure you are using. The head turning must be done slowly, free of any jerkiness. If you are getting good results with this, you can move lateral to the posterior angle of the ribs and even to the edge of the scapula and using a broader surface of your elbow and forearm, move the tissue from rib 1 down to rib 5 while she is doing the same head turning and focused breathing.

This technique would also be good in conjunction with the lumbar fascia and paraspinal fascia techniques in Chapter 8. It would be helpful to make at least one sweep down the length of the erectors after you have done this work just to connect the head

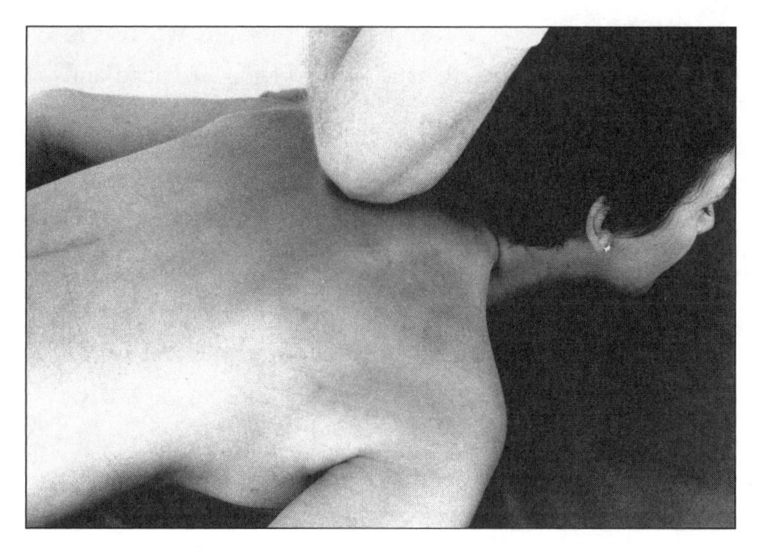

Figure 11.7

and neck with the low back via the fascial system. Work down the erectors several inches at a time. Pause occasionally to have the client breathe. When finishing this technique with the long pass down the erectors, you do not need to have the client turn her head.

> If the neck is extremely tight, have the client turn her head to tolerance, sink gently, wait for a softening, and then ask for movement through range of motion.

The Work: Treatment for Cervical Whiplash

Client Position: Prone, with head turned one way or the other

1. Place elbow point in the lamina groove starting at C7.

2. Apply pressure into the ribs and have client breathe into the point of contact.

3. Glide slowly down to maintain pressure, whereas at the same time, the client is slowly lifting her head and turning it to the other side.

4. Repeat up to three times on each side.

5. Move lateral to the posterior angle of the ribs and even to the edge of the scapula.

6. Make one sweep down the length of the erectors to connect the head and neck.

7. Pause and work the erectors when necessary.

Cervical Spine

These techniques are for your chronic neck clients, especially those with cervical kyphosis or even reverse cervical curve. It is useful to take a look at a lateral x-ray view of the client's cervical spine to ascertain the degree of kyphosis and curvature in the spine before proceeding with this technique. Figures 11.8–11.11 show the therapist using a prone pillow, which is a common device available from many medical or massage supply stores. Many body workers have massage tables that have very sophisticated face holders for this type of work. You do not need to run out and buy a prone pillow if your table is already equipped with a face cradle. However, the prone pillow is well-liked because it is so supportive of the head and shoulders, and makes the application of deep anterior pressure to the cervical spine easy to accomplish with minimum discomfort to the client. It is recommended before beginning this work to place the client in the face cradle and slowly compress her head or her shoulders to see where her point of discomfort is with the position of the face cradle. If her discomfort can be relieved by the use of rolled up towels, face cloths, props, or whatever, then go ahead and proceed. If the client is not comfortable, even with just

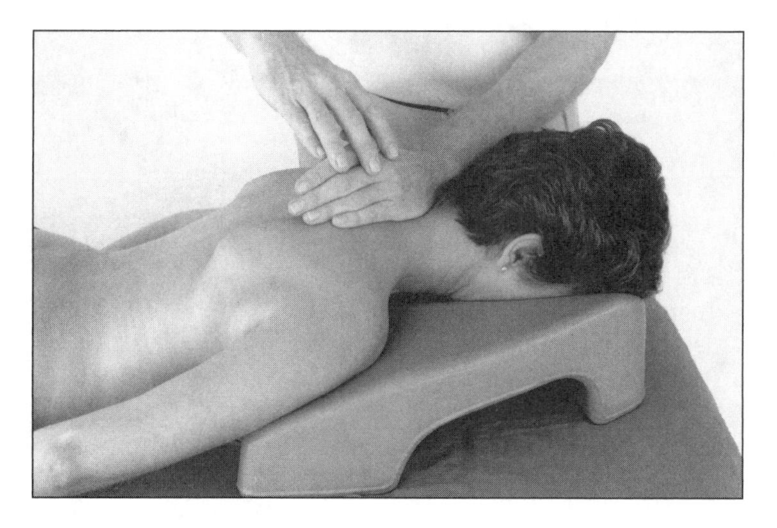

Figure 11.8

a slight amount of pressure, it is recommended to purchase one of these prone pillows before attempting this technique. Make sure that the client's forehead and frontal bone is well positioned over the top portion of the prone pillow or your face cradle, and check when you press the neck that her throat does not compress into the table or choke her slightly. Also for large-breasted women, you will need to place a pillow under their rib cage to help support them and minimize discomfort when you begin to compress the thoracic spine.

With the client comfortably positioned as in Figure 11.8, gently take the heel of your hand or the edge of the hypothenar eminence below your little finger and press down gently on the mid cervicals working all the way down to T4. Compression is directly on top of the spinous processes, and start very slowly and gradually build up the pressure. Then gently place your thumbs on top of the transverse processes from the second cervical vertebra, again down to the fourth thoracic, and compress those slightly anteriorly. Begin to assess which of the vertebrae are rotated by making a mental note of each vertebra and its transverse process, whether one side is higher than the other. As you compress gently over the spinous or transverse processes, ask

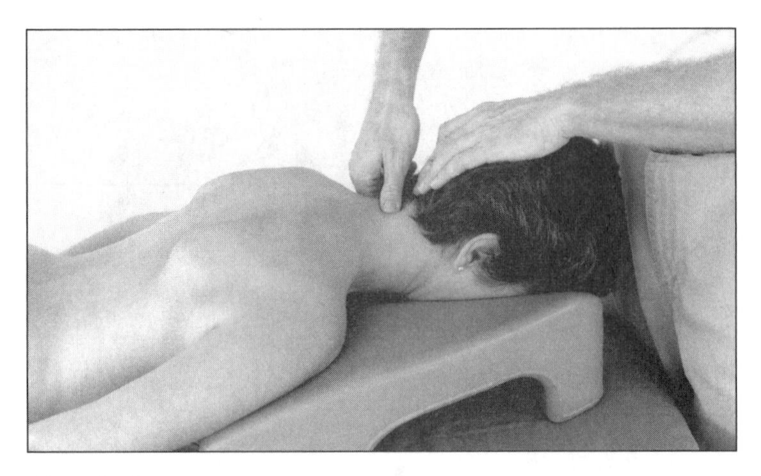

Figure 11.9

the client if there are any tender points. You may want to hold those tender points until she feels a relief from the tenderness. Repeat this process slowly with each vertebra once or twice all the way down to the fourth thoracic.

Next, use your elbow or thumbs, as shown in Figure 11.9, over the transverse processes and the posterior angle of the ribs moving from C7-T10. Make a gliding motion, like what the therapist's fingertips are doing in Figure 11.10, and in this way, gently warm up the larger planes of fascia and support structures of the neck. With your thumb or knuckle, apply pressure on the spinous process of C7 and slowly stretch the ligamentum nuchae from C7 to the occiput. This feels like you are moving along a very thin edge, so be careful not to apply too much pressure and slip off. The ligamentum nuchae is a highly specialized structure, and in a lateral view looks more like a sail on a boat with a centralized tendon posterior to the sail, and the anterior portions to the sail attaching to the spinous processes of the vertebrae. It is here where all the cervical fascia from the anterior to middle portions of the neck attach. You can repeat this process several times and even reverse the directions and go from the occiput down to C7.

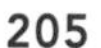

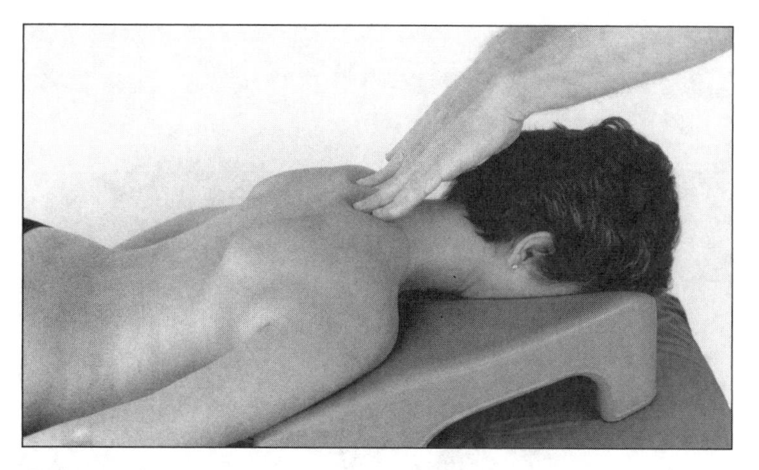

Figure 11.10

Then, search for trigger points on the occiput around the insertion of the trapezius, suboccipital triangle muscles, and large capitus muscles. Work bilaterally in the lamina groove from the occiput down to C7 searching for trigger points and fibrosity in the capitus muscles. You can work the areas of fibrosity by cross-fibering them. This step is shown in Figure 11.11. The next step is to finish the whole sequence of work by motion testing the vertebrae once again as you did in step number one. This time you can feel free to apply even more anterior compression over specific vertebrae and covering a broader area like the whole cervical spine or the first three thoracic vertebrae. You may like to motion test the vertebrae very slowly at first, and then after two or three compressions, build up to a more deep sustained pressure. The important thing to remember is that the neck actually has its base at the level of the third thoracic vertebra, which makes the fifth cervical vertebra the apex of the cervical curve. Many x-rays will show that the vertebra most disturbed in cervical whiplash trauma is indeed the fifth cervical, so it is here that you want to apply specific compression in order to reintroduce proper cervical curvature. When you have completed the above sequence of work, place a cold pack for up to 20 minutes over the back of the client's neck and upper dorsals.

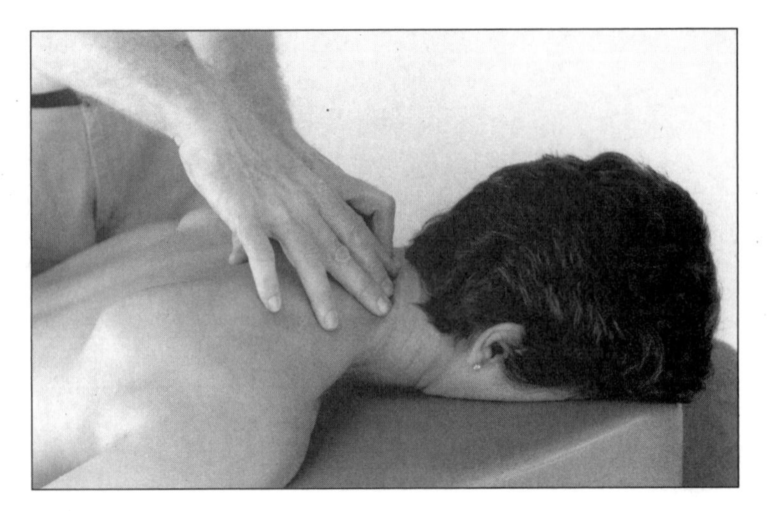

Figure 11.11

As an alternative, you can turn the client over, remove the prone pillow, roll up a towel, and place the cold pack over it. You can allow the client to rest and let the cold do its work. The use of hot packs is not particularly recommended when working with chronic neck conditions. After several minutes of tissue work, there is enough heat generated. After 15 to 20 minutes of this kind of work on the back of the neck, things will heat up quite a bit. Ice will be your best ally in reducing the pain and promoting healing in these types of cervical problems. As an alternative with this work, you can have the client lift her forehead off of the prone pillow about a half inch to an inch while you are working. Do this motion intermittently rather than constantly. This will help again rebuild the curvature.

> The more active a client is in his or her recovery, the better the outcome.

The Work: Cervical Spine

Client Position: Prone, with face support if necessary

1. Take heel of hand, fingertips, or thumbs and press down gently on the mid-cervicals working down to T4.

2. Compression is directly on top of the spinous processes.

3. Place one hand on transverse processes from the C2 to T4 and assess tender points or which of the vertebrae are rotated.

4. Use elbow or thumb over transverse processes from C7 to T10 making gliding motions.

5. Apply pressure on the spinous process of C7 and slowly stretch the ligamentum nuchae from C7 to occiput.

6. In addition, medial pressure can be added to the ligamentum nuchae.

7. Reverse direction, moving from occiput to C7.

8. Search and deactivate all trigger points.

9. Work bilaterally in the lamina groove searching for trigger points.

Suboccipitals

The suboccipitals lie deep in the posterior neck. They are frequently missed by therapists because they lie so deep. These muscles are named rectus capitus posterior major/minor and oblique capitus superior/inferior. Check your anatomy book and become familiar with this triangle of muscles. Specifically, the rectus capitis posterior minor attaches at the nuchal line of the occiput and originates at the atlas or C1. The rectus capitus posterior major inserts on the inferior aspect of the nuchal line and attaches at the axis or spinus process of C2. The oblique capitis superior attaches between the nuchal lines of the occiput and transverse process of C1. Last, the oblique capitis inferior attaches on the transverse process of C1 and the spinous process of C2. They are responsible for little movements of the head like nodding yes or no and rotating the head to the same side. The oblique capitis superior is responsible for lateral flexion.

The client is supine, and you are standing at the side of the table. Place your knuckle inferior to the mastoid process as seen in Figure 11.12. Sink deeply and begin a deep and very slow glide to the midline or external occipital protuberance. You want to really drop in with your vector anterior and superior to affect these muscles. Running too superficially will only affect the attachments along the occiput like the trapezius, the capitis muscles, and so on. You want to go deep to these. Sink incrementally, and the client will let you know when you are in an area of tenderness or discomfort. These attachments are generally very tender but welcome the work. Once you have treated the line along the occiput drop down inferiorly and repeat the process again, this time affecting the muscles on C2. Treat any trigger points along the way.

These muscles are deep to all neck muscles and require a special vector that is anterior and up.

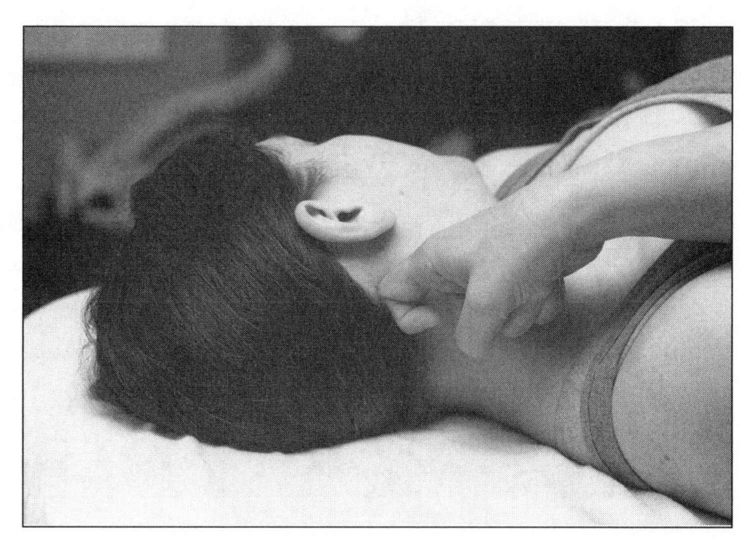

Figure 11.12

The Work: Suboccipitals

Client Position: Supine

1. Place knuckle inferior to the mastoid process.
2. Sink deeply and begin a deep and slow glide to the midline.
3. Repeat this process, again starting inferior to the mastoid process one finger width to start on C2.
4. Be sure to drop in and stay under the occiput, but snug to the bone.

Temporalis Fascia

As with some of the earlier techniques, the client is side lying, and her head should be supported with a pillow. This is an excellent way of working to free the tissue around the TMJ and the neck.

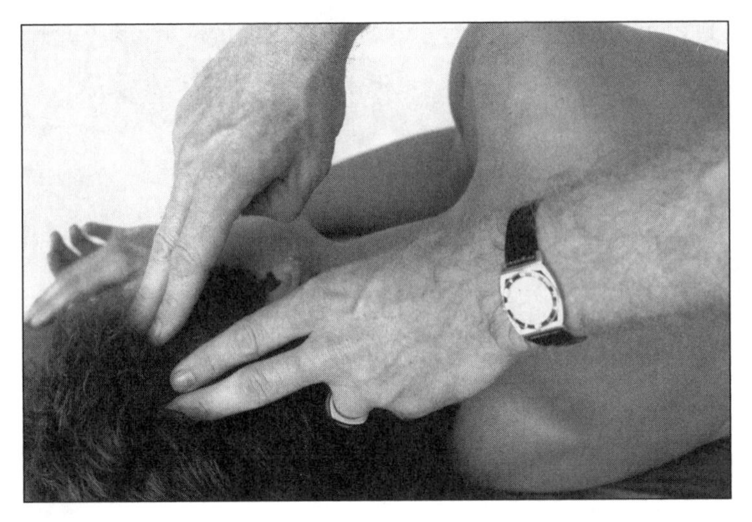

Figure 11.13

Place your fingertips directly above the ear on the coronal plane of the head. Refer to Figure 11.13. Then press into the head, and at the same time, begin spreading the tissue away from the midline. Move superiorly to the parietal ridge. Staying connected to the fascia will keep the hair from pulling. Only move one quarter to one half an inch at a time, and give the client ample opportunity to relax in between techniques. This work over the temporalis fascia can be repeated for several minutes, and you will feel a lot of heat and an occasional trigger point of release while you are spreading this fascia. It is recommended that you have the client clench her teeth and slowly stretch her mouth open from time to time while you are in the temporalis. This will really stretch that fascia as well as open up the TMJ. These releases for the external fasciae will also reflex into the pterygoid muscles inside the mouth and down into the masseter. This is a nice time to take a break to work the occipitofrontalis, scrub the scalp, and allow time for integration either before moving on to TMJ work or bringing your session to a close.

The Work: Temporalis Fasica

Client Position: Side lying, with knees flexed 45°

1. Place fingertips directly above the ear on the coronal plane.

2. Vector is into the tissues and up toward the head.

3. Wait for a release and move superiorly.

4. Move only one quarter to one half an inch at a time.

5. Give the client ample time to relax in between the technique.

6. Movements to ask for:

    - Clench teeth
    - Open mouth

Intraoral Techniques

Intraoral manual therapy is a very effective technique that works on the muscles inside and outside of the mouth. Clients who suffer from TMJ dysfunction, stress, and dental surgery find these techniques extremely beneficial. These techniques are intense, but safe, and require you to have good communication skills and stay mindful of autonomic activation. Gloves are worn at all times. Another thing to be mindful of is any latex allergies or use latex free gloves.

Palpation of the Hard Palate (Figures 11.14 and 11.15)

Landmark: Groove between the upper teeth and the roof of the mouth.

Client: Supine or seated, with mouth open wide.

Therapist: Seated or standing.

Verbalization: Ask client to lengthen the back of the neck.

Action: With index finger applying firm pressure on the roof of the mouth, attempt to spread the maxilla laterally. Stay off the soft palate. Hold the client's head firmly with your other hand. Watch for sympathetic activation.

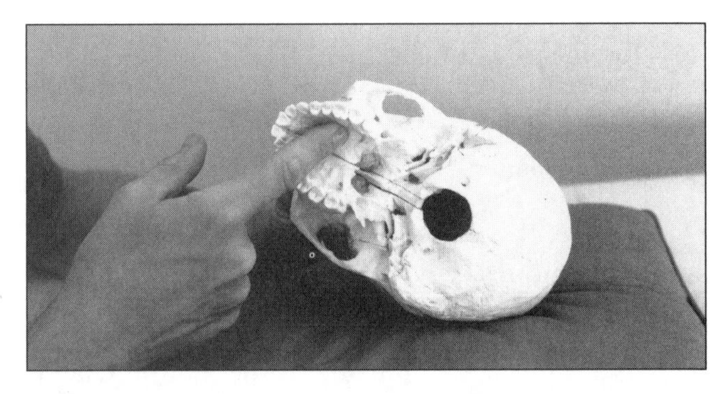

Figure 11.14

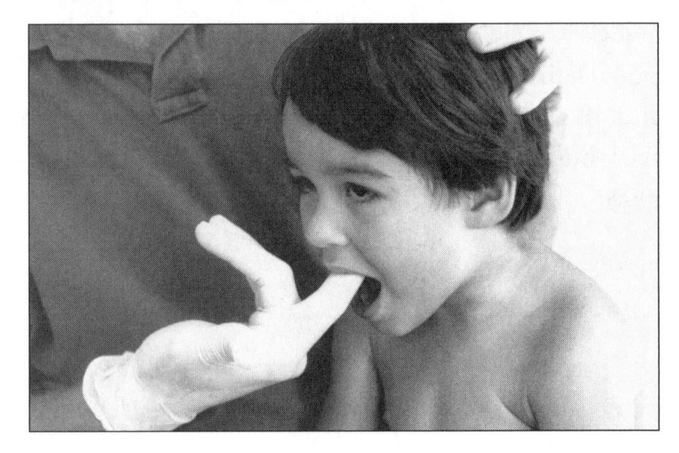

Figure 11.15

Release of the Masseter Muscle (Figures 11.16 and 11.17)

Landmark: Coronoid process of the mandible; lateral surface of the ramus.

Client: Supine or seated, with mouth open wide.

Therapist: Seated or standing.

Verbalization: Ask client to open wider and gently close.

Action: (1) Insert index finger between cheek and teeth until palpating muscle. (2) Wedge finger in the superior, posterior portion of the masseter, and ask for movement. Wait for the tissue to soften.

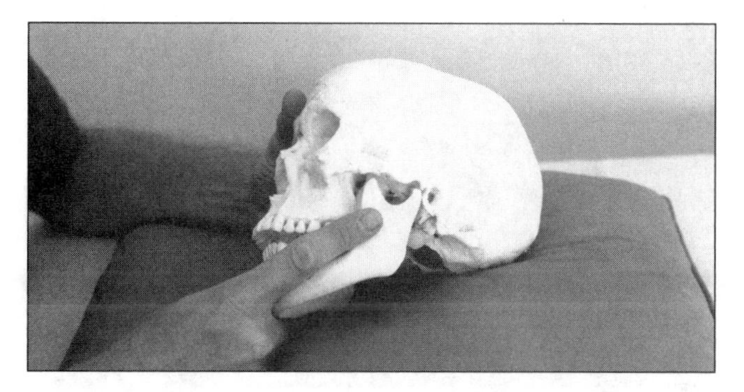

Figure 11.16

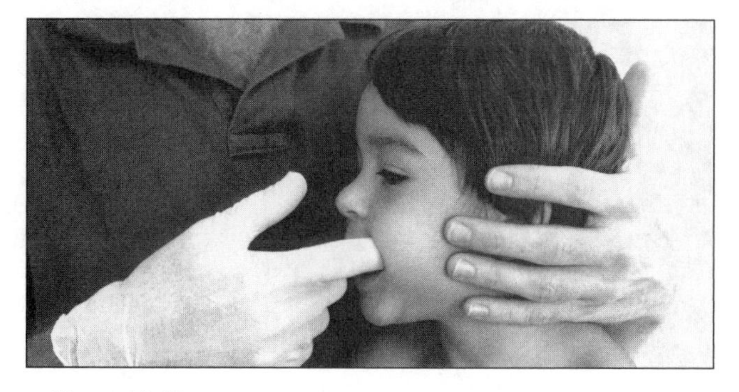

Figure 11.17

Release of the Medial Pterygoid (Figures 11.18 and 11.19)

Landmark: Medial surface of the ramus of the mandible.

Client: Supine or seated, with mouth open wide.

Therapist: Seated or standing.

Verbalization: (1) Ask patient to bite down gently, then slowly open mouth wide. (2) Keep breathing.

Action: (1) With index finger, follow upper inside gum-line back, just behind the upper molars. Apply steady pressure at superior attachment of the medial pterygoid. (2) Follow lower inside gum-line back, just behind the lower molars, to the angle of the ramus.

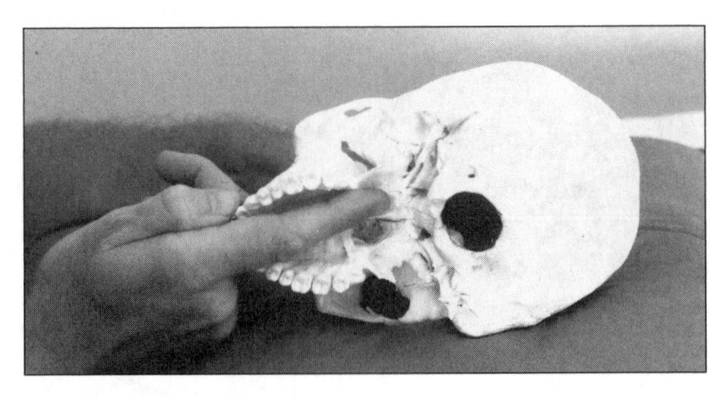

Figure 11.18

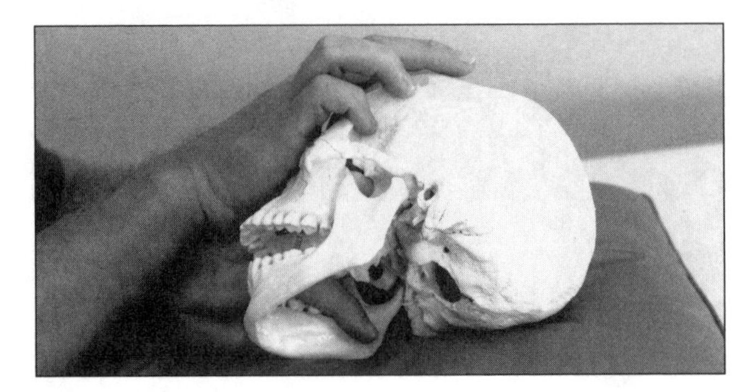

Figure 11.19

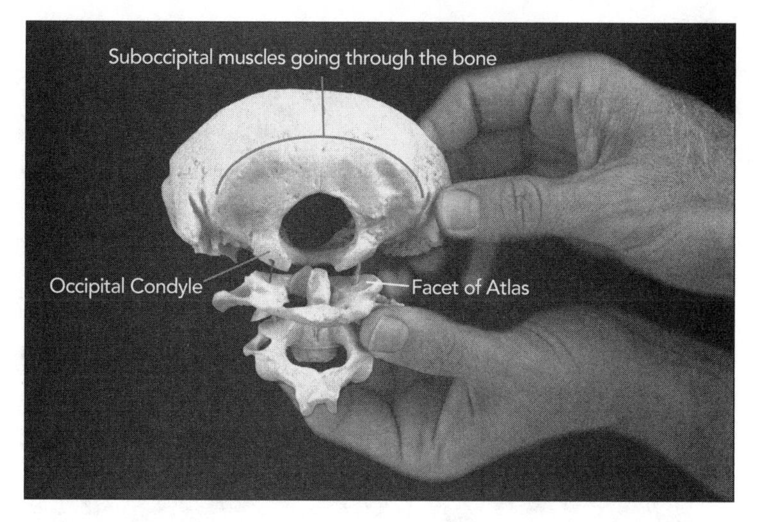

Figure 11.20

Atlas-Occiput Space

One of the nicest effects of these atlas-occiput space (AOS) explorations is how it settles the entire autonomic nervous system. This is the principal reason they are used in clinical practice. The point of contact is with the tips of the middle fingers (or others that are a better fit for the individual) of the practitioner in the AOS between the occiput and the second cervical vertebra. In this position, the practitioner's fingers are in contact with the superior cervical sympathetic ganglion. In addition, the fascia and muscle fibers of the suboccipital triangle actually go through the occiput and insert on the dura mater that covers the brain. This fascia is located just above the foramen magnum as shown in Figure 11.20. Thus, the AOS palpation skills are exceedingly important.

Variation 1

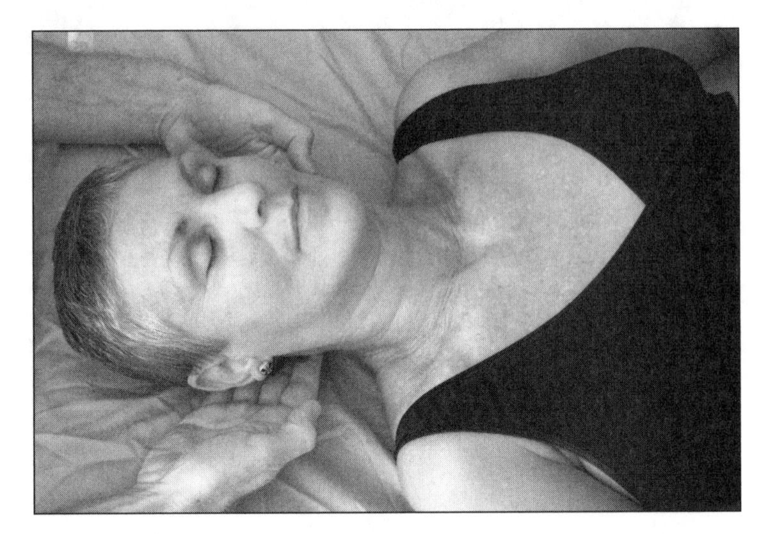

Figure 11.21

a. The client is supine in these explorations. The client's knees are flexed and resting together without any tension. If for some reason, the client's AOS is not responsive, then try having the client's legs straight out with a pillow under the knees.

b. The first step is to get the practitioner's hands together into a proper position as shown in Figure 11.21. The practitioner initial exploration is to slide his hands under the top of the client's neck with the pads of the pinky and ring fingers contacting the space of the suboccipital triangle of muscles and squama of the occiput. The rest of the finger pads are in the nape of the neck. The practitioner senses that whole area before getting more specific.

c. One important palpation skill in the AOS is to notice if there is any lymph edema there. It has a sense of the tissue being thick and spongy, as if filled with too much fluid. This is usually the result of congestion from a whiplash injury or other types of neck or head injuries. Dr. Sutherland was in the habit of always making sure the lymphatic ducts were open in the neck and thoracic outlet area when he worked with the cranium. The practitioner must help drain the lymph before proceeding further, or refer the client for lymph drainage if you notice such congestion in the AOS.

Variation 2

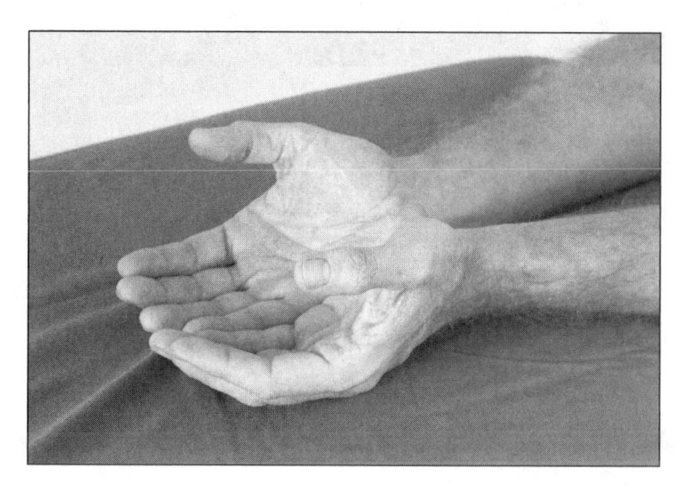

Figure 11.22

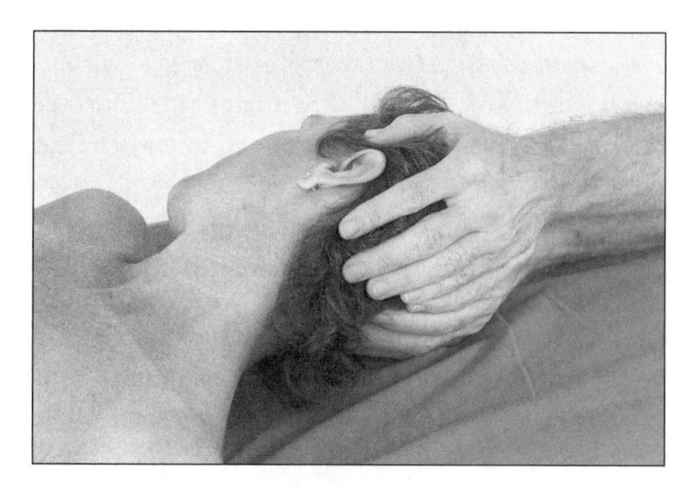

Figure 11.23

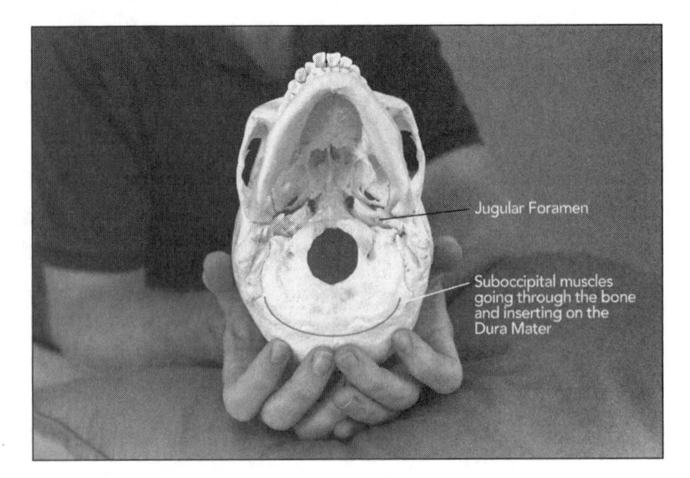

Figure 11.24

a. The practitioner lifts the client's head gently and rests it comfortably in his hands. The practitioner's ring and little fingers slightly overlap in such a way that the edges of the middle fingers (or depending on the size of the practitioner's hands, the index fingers) come together. Please study Figures 11.22, 11.23, and 11.24 for the precise finger positioning.

b. When placing the hands in this way under the client's head, the whole cranium of the client is cradled more or less in the medial aspects of the palms of the practitioner's hands. The tips of the middle fingers are used to discover the space between the occiput and the second cervical vertebra C2. This is the center of the AOS. The atlas (C1) has no spinous process, and consequently there is a gap between the occiput and C2. The pads of the middle fingers of the practitioner are resting against the client's occiput.

c. The practitioner softly cradles the client's head with full contoured contact of the client's cranium in the palms and hands of the practitioner.

d. Then the practitioner reorients and resynchronizes.

e. Then the practitioner slightly and gently curls the tips of the middle fingers back slightly as shown in Figure 11.25. This moves the client's chin ever so slightly into extension. If the client's neck is too stiff, the chin and cranium will not go into a slight extension. This is no problem, and the practitioner must not attempt to force or push the clients head into extension. It is recommended that the client have some soft tissue work done on her neck before the next cranial session.

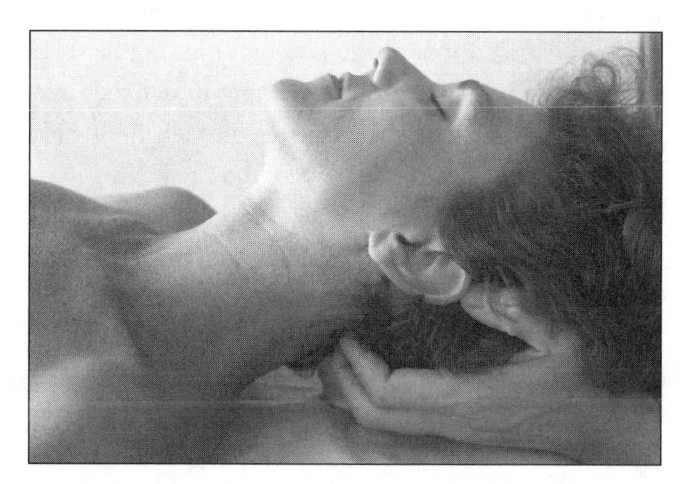

Figure 11.25

a. Next, the tips of the middle fingers begin to wedge slightly into the AOS with more firmness. Again, there is a need to listen locally and globally for a minute or so during each stage of this process. This is because the muscles of the suboccipital triangle will soften gradually and usually soften one side at a time, and the fluid body and autonomic nervous system need time to get in register with the other layers. Consequently, the practitioner must keep accommodating to the motion of the client's head when the soft tissue relaxes on both sides. In other words, as the tissue softens, the practitioner takes up the slack in the tissues by allowing his fingertips to move up into the AOS without excessive pressure, but staying at the edge of any barriers encountered.

Variation 3

a. While cradling the AOS with the tips of the middle fingers, a figure eight may be explored through the fluid body of the practitioner into the suboccipital triangle of the client in the tempo of primary respiration. In other words, the practitioner begins to move his whole fluid body very subtly like a snake writhing or dancing in a figure eight. That motion translates through the hands of the practitioner into the AOS of the client. The practitioner periodically stops his motion and listens locally and out to the horizon. The basic motion in the fluid body is a spiral, and the figure eight helps to amplify the therapeutic properties of the spiral.

b. The motions described above in terms of the figure eight and tractioning are done with the whole hands and fluid body of the practitioner, not just the fingertips.

Variation 4

a. Gently laterally spread the middle fingers by moving the elbows together. This influences the jugular foramen and relieves pressure on the vagus nerve and jugular vein.

Variation 5

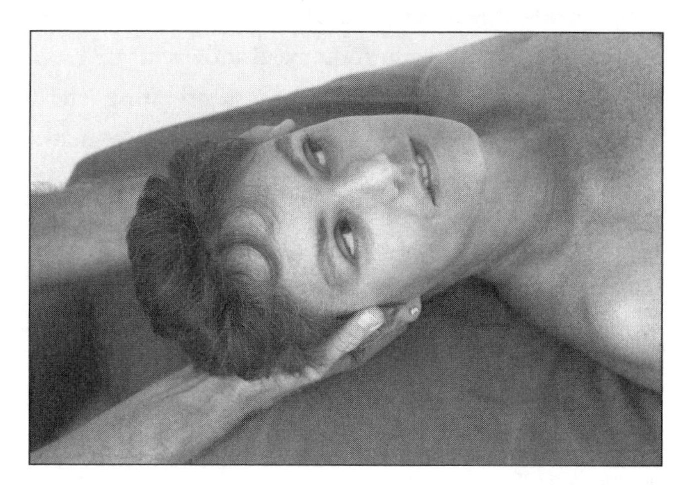

Figure 11.26

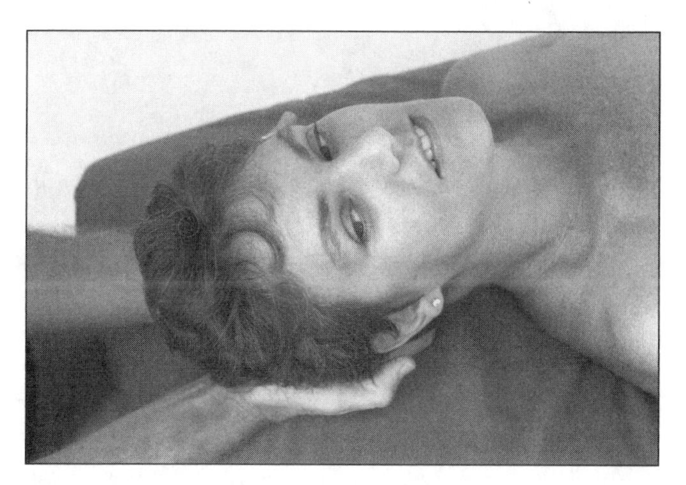

Figure 11.27

a. This AOS exploration involves the orienting reflex and the head righting reflex. All of the AOS explorations have the ability to recalibrate visual and auditory attention to an external stimuli. This is a reflex located in the proprioceptors of the upper cervical spine and the cranial nerve nuclei including the fifth cranial nerve. The head righting reflex is associated with being able to rest one's visual gaze on the horizon. In addition, this same reflex is related to the ability to turn the head and orient to novel stimuli in the environment, which is the orienting reflex. Both of these reflexes are compromised with traumatic stress, and the head becomes separate from the body in terms of perception.

b. The practitioner asks the client to rotate her head to the left slowly and only a short distance of a couple of inches.

c. Repeat head turn to the left.

d. Now ask the client to look to the left and turn the head to the left as shown in Figure 11.26.

e. Repeat to the right.

f. Bring client's head to the center.

g. Now the practitioner asks the client to look right while the practitioner rotates the client's head to the left as shown in Figure 11.27. Note restrictions or motion barriers and stop when meeting a barrier and wait for it to soften.

h. Repeat the sequence to the opposite side.

i. This is a very powerful way to work and should not be attempted for several sessions and only if the above variations are ineffective.

Variation 6

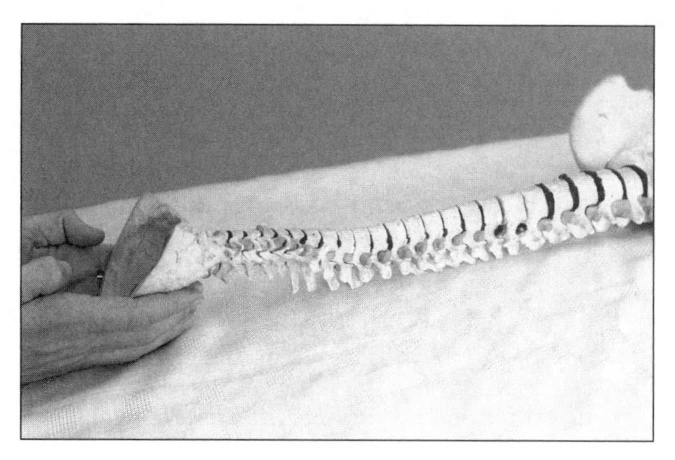

Figure 11.28

a. Place a microgram of traction on the occiput to explore the dura mater and any tension patterns it might be holding especially from whiplash injuries. This is a very delicate traction that is done for several seconds and then released. Figure 11.28 shows the position of the fingers on the occiput.

b. It can be repeated several times or until the practitioner senses he is at the sacral attachment of the dura mater. It is barely an intention to traction. The tractional force is measured in nanograms!

c. It is also helpful to visualize the dural tube with its denticulate ligaments and subarachnoid space full of cerebrospinal fluid. In addition, the blood vascular supply to the meninges can be visualized as if the dura was pink and red. See below for more detailed instructions.

Review of AOS Variations

Variation 1

The practitioner gets a sense of the whole area of the upper neck with his finger pads.

Variation 2

1. Client is supine with practitioner sitting at head of client.

2. Hands are positioned for an occiput cradle with middle fingers at AOS.

3. Pads on occiput, tips of fingers toward body of atlas in soft tissue.

4. Practitioner's middle fingers are slightly curled back toward the atlas in the soft tissue area.

5. Practitioner holds the head like a bowl of water and senses primary respiration.

Variation 3

1. Bring head into slight extension by slowly moving the whole head in a figure eight with the micromovement.

2. Motion test with a figure eight: slightly rotate head to right not more than a one quarter inch.

3. Side bend head to direction of ease, with micro motion.

4. Repeat sequences every 2 minutes while waiting in between.

5. Maximum three sequences.

6. Wait and sense opening and lengthening through soft tissue.

Variation 4

1. The practitioner gently brings his elbows closer together.

2. This exerts a lateral spreading of the fingers which influences the jugular foramen to open and soften.

Variation 5

1. Client moves eyes to right; practitioner turns head right several inches and back to midline. Repeat on left. Go slowly at the tempo of primary respiration.

2. Then have client look with her eyes to one side while rotating the head to the opposite side.

3. Repeat to the opposite side.

4. Repeat a maximum of three times or until opening and lengthening are sensed in the AOS and cervical spine down to the sacrum.

Variation 6

1. Visualize the dura mater and subarachnoid space that is filled with cerebrospinal fluid on the inside and attached to the vertebrae on the outside via the denticulate ligaments starting at the foramen magnum.

2. Offer a nanogram of traction for 15 to 30 seconds on the occiput.

3. Slowly count down the vertebrae from the first cervical all the way to the second sacral segment.

4. Relax intention and wait 15 to 30 seconds when noticing a tension or restriction in the dura mater. Practice moving attention out through the zones and back.

5. Let the dura mater soften before moving on or simply go around the restriction if it chooses to remain.

6. Repeat until sensing the dural tube attachment at the sacrum. In some clients, continue down to the feet to imagine the client's body becoming like seaweed.

7. Finally, fill the subarachnoid space and dura mater with a beautiful pink light from the cardiovascular system.

8. Caution must always be used with visualizations involving the inside of a client's body. The practitioner must be able to sense if the client is reacting to the visualization usually through a tissue contraction or the fluid body becoming tense. If softening and lengthening of the dura mater do not start occurring with a minute or two, then the practitioner must abandon the visualization.

Process

One of the common mistakes is for the practitioner to relax the fingertips whereas it is important to take up the slack as the suboccipital triangle softens as mentioned. In this way, the atlas can begin to reseat itself onto the occipital condyles, and a proper relationship along the whole suture line between the occiput and temporal bone can occur. Also, it is taught in the French Osteopathic Schools that the client's knees must be flexed for work in and around the AOS. It is recommended trying both ways with knees flexed and without, and see which is better for that client. Frequently, the clients go fast asleep when your fingers are engaged in the AOS, and consequently the knees must be well supported and without held tension in the legs if they are flexed.

When a client is really high toned sympathetically, if you start with an AOS exploration, it may make it much easier to sense the fluid body and tidal body. This is a judgment call on the part of the practitioner that requires skill and practice.

The biodynamic practitioner starts with the whole, and in the middle of a session, may move to more functional explorations if invited to do so. Nonetheless, every session begins and ends biodynamically. In other words, the best time to explore the AOS is in the middle of a session.

Summary

Contact is made with the superior cervical sympathetic ganglion in all the AOS variations. Trauma to the orienting reflex nerves may cause a person to have difficulty sensing her environment, which feels like an inability to easily turn the head or to rest attention on the horizon all the way to claustrophobic thinking and emotional breakdowns. This greatly interferes with the ability to perceive primary respiration from the horizon and back. It decreases one's ability to relate accurately with the environment, which is a hallmark of traumatic stress.

Finally, the occiput is the primary stress bone during a vaginal delivery. There are three typical intraosseous patterns imprinted in the occiput from birth. They are called shelving, telescoping, and torsion. During exploration with the AOS, as well as the transverse sinus in Chapter 17, it is possible to encounter these birth dynamics and normalize any intraosseous or interosseous stress imprinting from birth as long as the practitioner is synchronized with primary respiration.

CHAPTER 12

Releases for the Viscera

Mobilizing the Liver and Respiratory Diaphragm

This sequence of work is a very comprehensive treatment for the diaphragm, and also for a congested liver. Remember that you do not have to have a congested liver to get this treatment because it is primarily for the diaphragm. You can see in Figure 12.1 that the therapist has placed one hand on top of the other over the client's liver. She is lying on her left side with the knees drawn up and the head supported with a pillow. The first step is to bring your hands to a neutral position with no weight being added. The next step is to just follow the client's respiratory pattern, the rise and the fall as the diaphragm moves through inhalation and exhalation. Once you have an idea of her breath, you can begin the technique by following her exhalation and accentuating it greatly with several pounds of pressure, up to even 20 pounds of pressure. This compression is a straight medial compression of the ribs, liver, pleura, and lungs toward the spine. Do not hold her exhalation at its end point any longer than a second or two, as this can cause distress. Gradually relax your pressure as she inhales so that once again at the top part of her inhale, your hands are essentially feather light. The next step is to again follow the exhalation of the client, and this time your compression is both medial and inferior toward the pelvis. This helps move the diaphragm and pleura with an excellent stretch. Again you'll get to

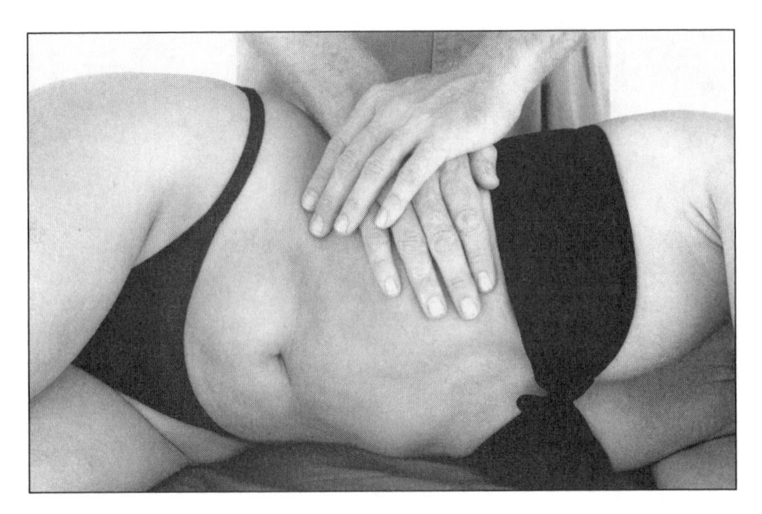

Figure 12.1

the end point of her exhalation and when you feel this, you want to let them inhale without restriction and rather than lifting your hands off of them, just gradually lighten the pressure but maintain contact.

The next step is to place your hands in a position beside one another as in Figure 12.2. Have the client take a deep breath, and again as she is exhaling, slowly begin to compress her ribs toward her spine. This time you want to imagine that you could roll her rib cage, as though you have hold of a cylinder, forward toward the xiphoid process. This is not to say that you are going to push the client in prone position, but rather it is as though your back thumbs are hooked on the posterior angle of the ribs or close to them, and your fingertips are around toward the sternum. The feeling is that you are rolling a cylinder in place while also placing compression toward the spine. This work feels very good to receive, especially afterward when a client has stood up. You can repeat this whole sequence of work three times, depending on the severity of the restriction of the diaphragm or the liver.

Many people, especially senior citizens who are on numerous prescription drugs, are causing their livers to work overtime. This

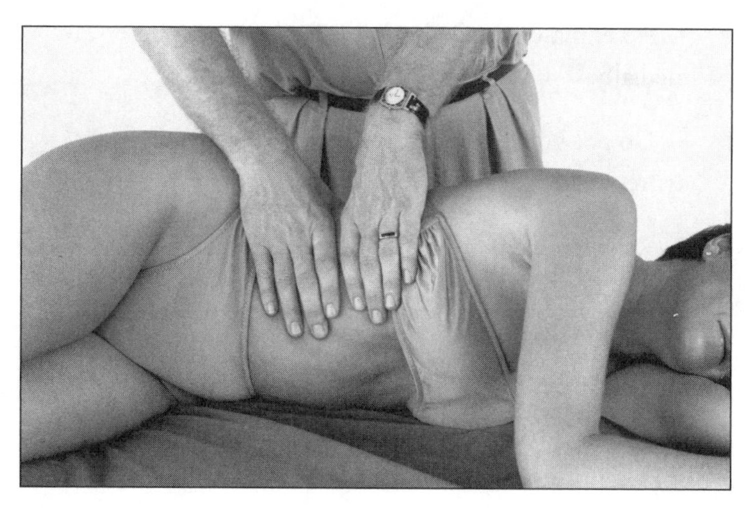

Figure 12.2

compression on the liver is a good way of exercising the liver and flushing the bile ducts. It is a common, easy thing to accomplish and very generic in its effect and certainly harmless to do it you are not sure of the technique. The client's respiration in this case is your guide, and it is important to not stress her by holding her exhalation more than several seconds at a time. The key is to pay attention to her breathing and know exactly when she is at the top of her inhale and the bottom of her exhale. Many students forget to direct the client's breath or get lost in the middle of the technique. Just take your hands off the client and ask her to breathe easy for a minute.

The Work: Mobilizing the Liver and Respiratory Diaphragm

Client Position: Side lying, on left side with knees flexed 45°

1. Place one hand on top of the other over the client's liver.
2. Bring hands to a neutral position with no weight.
3. Follow the client's respiratory pattern.

4. Accentuate the exhale with several pounds of pressure medially.

5. Do not hold longer than a second or two. May cause distress.

6. Relax pressure on the inhale.

7. Using feather light pressure, accentuate the inhalation.

8. Follow the exhalation and vector compression medially and inferiorly.

Respiratory Diaphragm and the Liver

These techniques are a very comprehensive way of working with both the respiratory diaphragm and the liver. The client sits with her pelvis slightly above her knees and her feet are slightly in front of her knees and are spread a hips-width apart. The client needs to be seated up straight with the arms down by the side. As you can see in Figure 12.3, the therapist's right hand is just below the costal arch and is pressing in slightly toward the midline of the body and also toward his back hand, which is placed very gently on the spine directly in a line with his front hand. This technique is done in two ways. The first is to have the client bend over very slightly with the head moving toward the knees perhaps a foot. Then take your right hand and hook your fingers underneath the costal arch, and they will come into contact with the respiratory diaphragm. Then have the client sit back up, and as she is sitting back up, lift the costal arch with several pounds of pressure, and this will stretch the diaphragm. You can repeat this procedure several times moving your hand just lateral to the xiphoid process. Then you can move more laterally off the costal arch several inches until you get almost to the side or the coronal plane of the trunk. You can repeat this procedure two or three times on each side. You may like to twist and turn the trunk

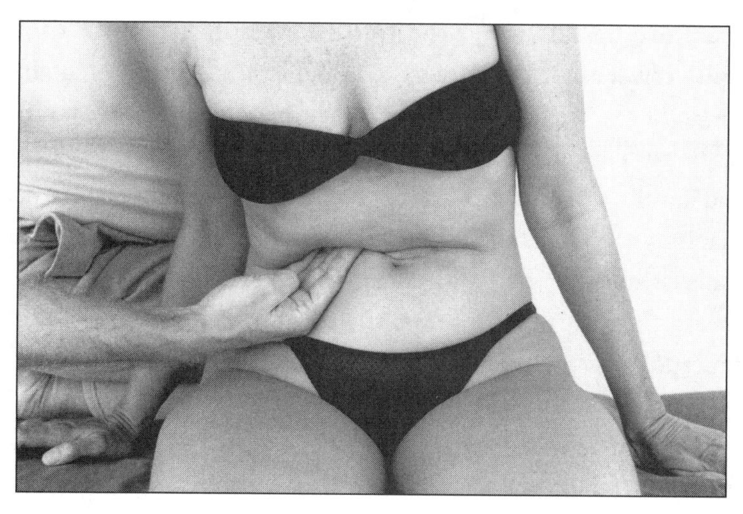

Figure 12.3

while having a client in this position. That means, that while you are lifting on the costal arch, you are also twisting her trunk from side to side and turning it as well as side-bending it.

Figure 12.4 shows the therapist working on the liver. The starting position for this technique is the same as the one above. With the client in the seated position, take your right hand and place it several inches lateral from the xiphoid process toward the liver. When the client begins to bend forward, about 12 to 15 inches, have her stop, and this time instead of hooking your fingers under the costal arch, press your fingers as far back toward the posterior abdominal wall as you can. The point of entry with your fingers cannot be directly below the costal arch but rather several inches below the costal arch. When the client bends forward and you press your hands back, you are taking up all the slack in the skin and superficial fascia. Therefore, you will run out of room real quick unless you put enough slack into the abdomen because you want your hand to go back as far as it can. Now that your hand has gone several inches back toward the posterior abdominal wall, have the client side-bend her body to the right, and very slowly with as broad a contact as you can with all the pads of your fingertips, lift up into the liver. Normally the tissue of the liver feels very dense and somewhat tight. The idea here is to mobilize the right and left triangular ligaments that attach the liver to the respiratory diaphragm. It is not unusual at all for clients who have had injuries and are short of breath or have restrictions around their diaphragm to have these restrictions reflex into their liver. Thus some clients will report nutritional or digestive problems along with their orthopedic problems. You can repeat this process two or three times moving your hand several inches lateral. It is recommended removing your hand after each time you palpate the lover, having the client sit back up straight and with you placing your hand very lightly over the costal arch, ask her to take a breath into where you just worked. Alternately what you may like to do when your hand is lifting the liver, is to ask the client to take a breath around the point of contact. It must be done slowly.

Respiratory Diaphragm and Stomach

This work is continuation of the work on the liver and diaphragm. In this case, move over the left side of the body. That is because

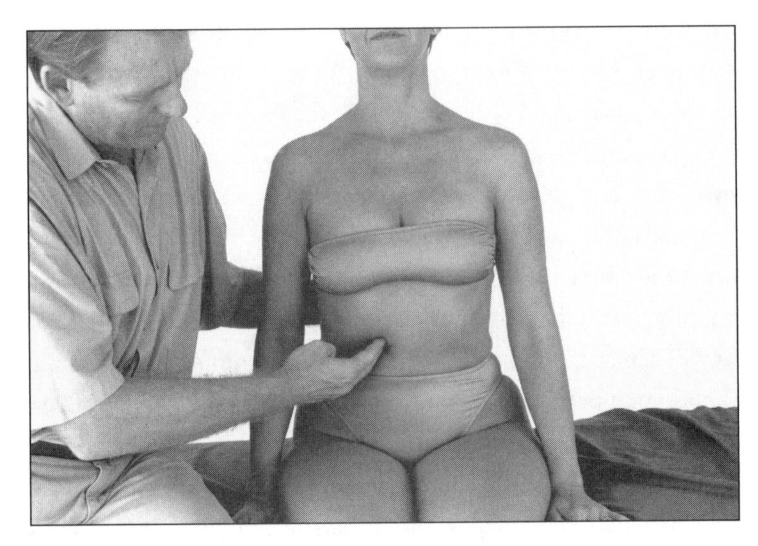

Figure 12.4

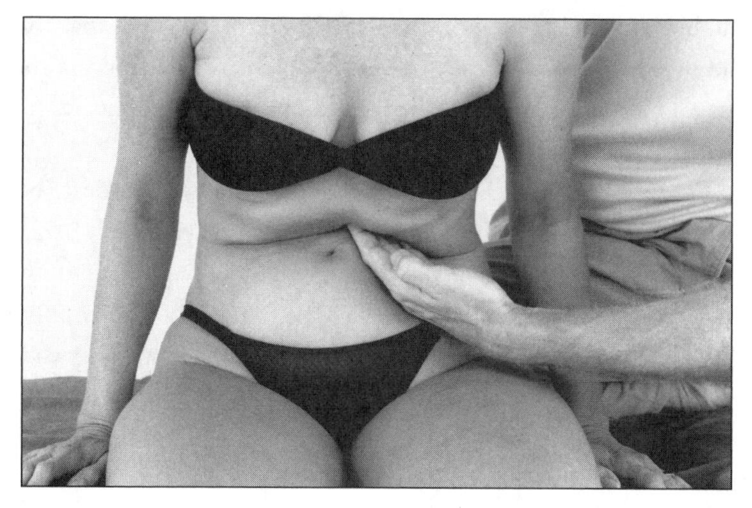

Figure 12.5

the stomach occupies a space just to the left of the midline of the abdomen. You can see in Figure 12.5 that the therapist has taken his left hand and once again, hooked his fingers under the costal arch. At this point, the procedure is the same as before: have the client bend forward slightly, while at the same time you are hooking your fingers underneath the costal arch. Then have the client sit up straight, while at the same time you lift the costal arch with 5 to 10 pounds of pressure. This lift of the costal arch and opening of the diaphragm will also give the stomach an opportunity to stretch and lift. The stomach can be depressed down lower into the abdomen. The stomach is depressed for any number of reasons, especially overeating and stomach ulcers as well as lack of proper exercise. The stomach is suspended off of the respiratory diaphragm by the phrenico gastric ligament. Once again, it is a technique that will not only increase respiratory function by opening the diaphragm but also stretch the stomach and its ligament attachment to the diaphragm. In applying this technique, the walls of the stomach in clients that have had ulcers will scar down and cause adhesions. This is a very good stretch for any client who has had a history of ulcers, and you will be surprised at how many clients do not remember that they had ulcers 15 to 20 years ago. Many adolescents have ulcers that cause adhesions, and these adhesions can be the cause of nutritional problems and digestive problems later in life.

Figure 12.6 shows the therapist working bilaterally as described in an earlier technique. The approach is to position your body behind the client and place both of your hands under the costal arch. In this case, both of the therapist's hands are just to the left of the midline of the body in the position of the stomach and hiatal opening where the esophagus comes through the diaphragm. This technique can be employed for those clients that experience a hiatal hernia from time to time, as well as those clients who are chronically short of breath. The starting position for this technique is with the client seated straight up. The photograph shows the position as to how far forward you want the client to bend when you are doing the technique. Allow your fingers to go more posteriorly toward the back, and while the client is bending forward, you then allow your fingers to lift up into that cardia, which is the hiatal opening. This is an area of much neurological innervation. The vagus nerve is here along with the phrenic nerve, and it is very sensitive to this type of mobilization. Another thing that you can do with the client while in this position is to take your fingers and move them down toward the umbilicus at the same depth and pressure while the client is lifting up. This is also a very good counter stretch for the stomach and the diaphragm. As before, it is vital to have the client breathe into the point of contact while you are in either the stomach, diaphragm, or liver. It is also of equal importance that the client be given a break after each lift is done. Gently place your hand over where you just worked and your opposite hand in the back over the floating ribs, and ask the client to breathe very slowly and gently into both of your hands. After the client does this two or three times, then you can move on and attempt the technique again if necessary.

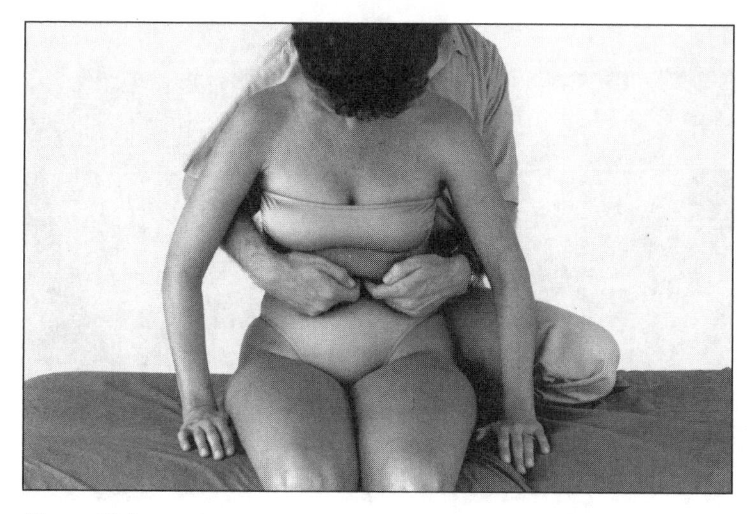

Figure 12.6

Bladder Ligaments under the Pubic Symphysis

This is a wonderful release, especially for those clients that have chronic low back pain that is not responding to traditional therapy. There are somato-visceral and visceral-somato reflexes that can be at play here. That is to say that a tight quadratus and an over-involvement of the lumbar fascia can have reflexes into the organs of the pelvis floor. Likewise, someone with a bladder infection or other visceral problems can reflex into the soft tissue of the low back. This is a favorite release to do in conjunction with the psoas release because it really opens up the floor of the pelvis and helps to lengthen the lumbar fascia by means of these reflexes. You can see in Figure 12.7 that the therapist has placed his hand palm down on the client's abdomen. The tips of his fingers are on the superior edge of the pubic bone since he has compressed his hand about an inch into the abdomen. Start right on the midline of the pubic symphysis and allow your hand now to sink even further into the abdomen as though you were going to try to get your fingertips underneath the pubic bone, which in fact you are attempting to do.

Once you feel you are just slightly under the pubic symphysis

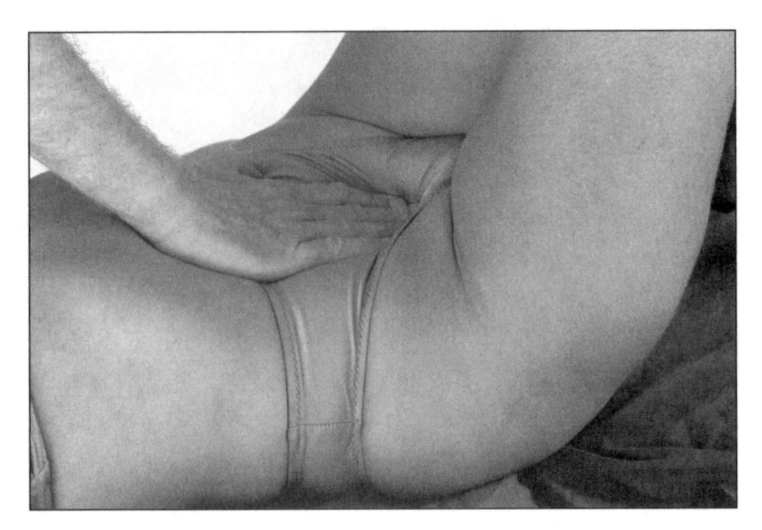

Figure 12.7

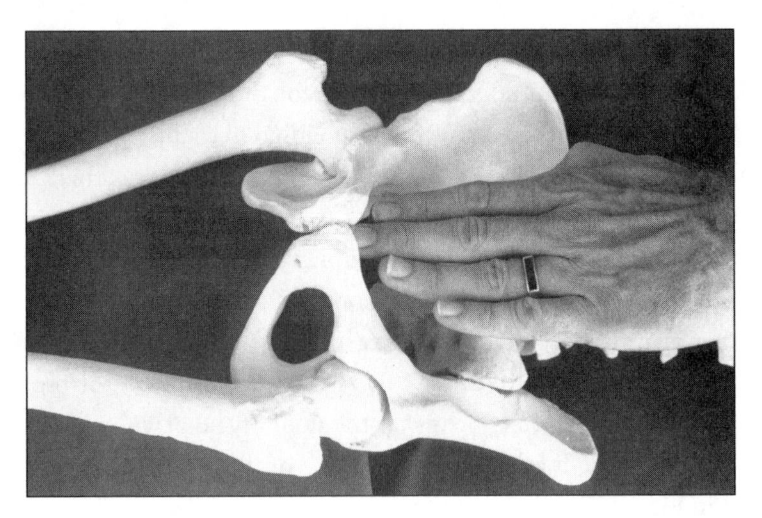

Figure 12.8

(Figure 12.8), and you know the tissue will be very taunt at this point, hold your compression and ask the client if she feels any pain. There are several trigger points here on the midline and just lateral that you will be looking for. If the client reports tenderness, then hold the point until you feel it soften and gradually back off and just slide your hand a quarter of an inch to one side or the other and repeat this procedure. It is best to start with your hand fully an inch above the pubic symphysis as you compress and search, so that you take up the slack of the superficial fascia of the abdomen and not the tight tissue around the pubic symphysis. That way when you get your fingertips underneath the pubic bone, you will have a more accurate feeling at your fingertips for what is tight and what is loose. The pressure you are using is anywhere from a couple of pounds to maybe 10 or 15 pounds. Always do this in conjunction with the client's permission and an eye on her face. She will tell you very definitely when you are on a sore point and when you are not. The important thing is to have a sense of softening, and the client connecting with this same sense of release or ease from her discomfort. If there are significant restrictions, then you cannot expect them to all go away with one treatment. You should know that there are numerous ligaments and a lot of neurological activity around the bladder and its attachment to the underside of the pubic bone.

It is for this reason that it is highly recommended to get out a good anatomy book and take a look at a cross section of the pelvic floor, and particularly the organs of the urogenital system. The key to this technique is in putting enough slack into the pubic symphysis and going around it. It will be much too painful. Just place your hand palm down with your fingertips an inch or so above the pubic symphysis, make your posterior compression, and then your inferior glide under the pubic bone will be much easier. You can also have the client assist by having her lift her tailbone very slightly toward the ceiling or moving her tailbone toward the table. Remember also to have the client bring her knees up with her feet slightly spread so that her legs rest comfortably without tension against each other. This puts slack into the rectus abdominis and makes your work much easier. Some clients cannot rest their knees together, so gently tie a strap around their knees, and this will take the tension out of their legs and abdomen. Finally, it is important to have the client breathe into the area you have worked on. You may need to cue this by gently placing your hand over the area you just completed.

The Work: Bladder Ligaments under Pubic Symphysis

Client Position: Supine, with knees bent, use strap if necessary

1. Place your palm down on client's belly with tips of fingers on superior edge of pubic bone.
2. Gently and mindfully allow fingers to sink posteriorly as if trying to get fingers under the client's pubic bone.
3. When taut tissue is felt, ask client if she feels any pain.
4. If tenderness is reported, hold point until a softening is felt.
5. Once a softening is felt, gently back off and move either medially or laterally to search for other tender areas.
6. Movements to ask for are:
   - Move tailbone toward the ceiling
   - Move tailbone toward the table

Bladder Ligaments between the Bladder and the Umbilicus

These techniques are a continuation of the bladder release just completed on the preceding page. They can also be done by themselves when the bladder and floor of the pelvis is too sensitive to palpate. The bladder is suspended from the umbilicus by three ligaments. There is a central ligament and two lateral ligaments that are just about a half inch lateral from the midline. Use your thumbs as in Figure 12.9, or as the therapist's fingertips as in Figure 12.10. At the beginning, place your thumbs just above the pubic symphysis on the midline and allow them to sink into the rectus abdominis, which is where those bladder ligaments are located. They are actually on the posterior surface of the rectus abdominus. Once you compress the rectus very slowly, attempt to feel this ligament that is like a tiny string coming down from the umbilicus. Regardless of whether you feel the ligament or not, you can do the technique that is accomplished by gliding your thumbs an inch or two at a time moving from inferior to superior toward the umbilicus. Ask the client to lift her tailbone slightly as well as tuck it down toward the table. This is very beneficial for opening up the floor of the pelvis with these techniques.

Once you get up toward the umbilicus on the midline, then start back again slightly above the pubic symphysis—this time with your thumbs or fingers just slightly lateral of the midline, and again work your way up toward the umbilicus several inches at a time. You can repeat this work up to three times on the midline and lateral to it. You will be surprised at how many clients have had exploratory surgeries, laparoscopies, hysterectomies, appendectomies, and other surgical procedures in their pelvic floor and abdomen that will benefit from this work. There are so many adhesions that form in the peritoneum and pelvis from surgeries and intestinal problems. This work has a very freeing sensation, especially when the client stands up after the work. Two things are important to remember. The first is that after each time you work in the abdomen, place your hand over where you just worked and ask the client to take a slow easy breath into your hand. The second thing to remember is that when the client stands up, once again place your hands over the front and back sides of the abdomen and lumbars and ask her to relax her abdomen into your hands as well as breathe in between your two hands. There needs to be some constant reminder for the client to breathe into her belly especially if she has a history of trauma.

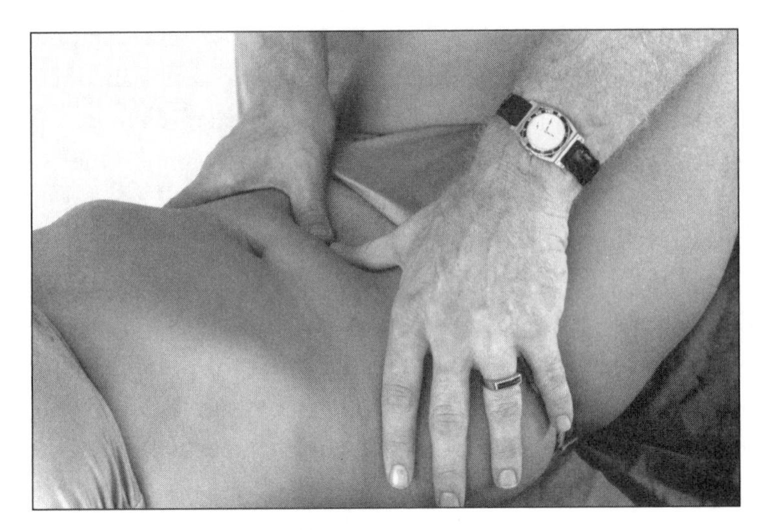

Figure 12.9

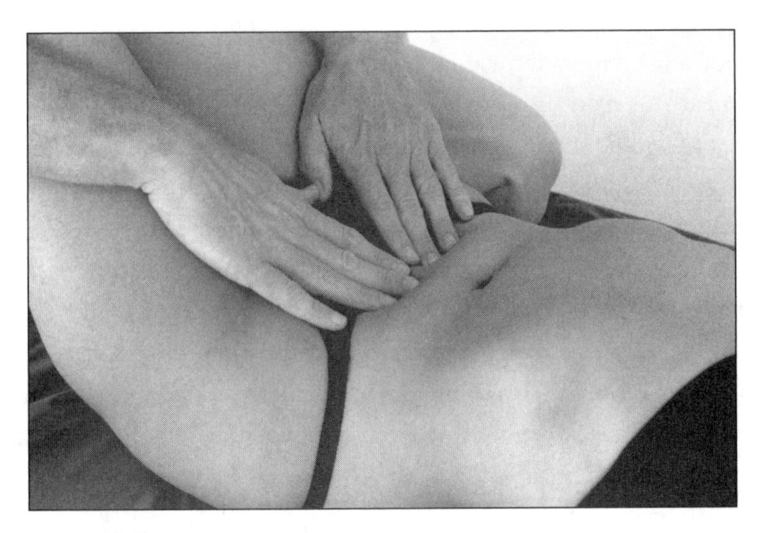

Figure 12.10

The Work: Bladder Ligament between Bladder and Umbilicus

Client Position: Supine, with knees flexed, use strap if necessary

1. Facing the client's head, place thumbs or fingertips just above the pubic symphysis on the midline, allowing thumbs to sink into the rectus abdominus.
2. Feeling for the ligaments, gently compress posteriorly into the belly.
3. Glide superiorly toward the umbilicus searching for tender areas.
4. Repeat the work coming back to the pubic symphysis and move laterally and repeat.
5. Repeat up to three times.
6. Movements to ask for:
   - Lift and tuck the tailbone
   - Breath into the belly

Iliacus and Cecum

This work is a valuable technique for working a part of the illio-psoas that very often is overlooked. Specifically it has to do with releasing the two ligamentus attachments to the cecum, which as you may recall from your anatomy, is the lower part or pouch of the ascending colon where the illiocecal valve joins the small intestines with the large intestines. In addition, this technique is also good for releasing the iliacus muscle, and as such, its fascial continuity with the adductors of the lower leg. You can see in Figure 12.11 and Figure 12.12 that the therapist's fingertips start the point of

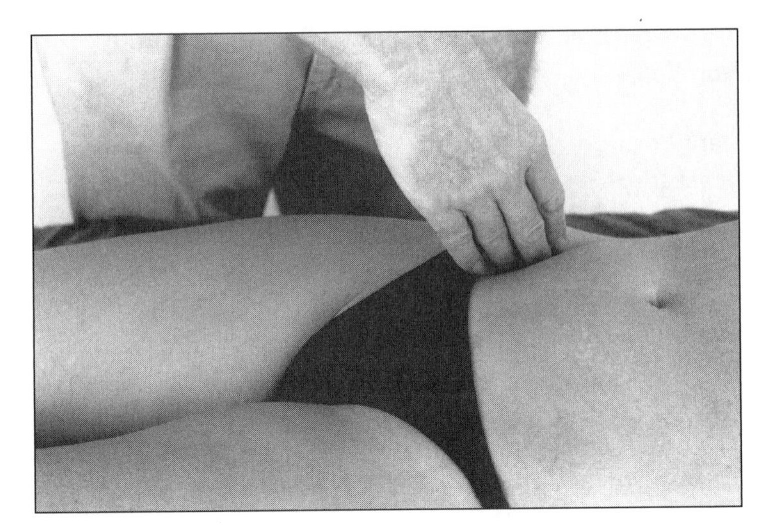

Figure 12.11

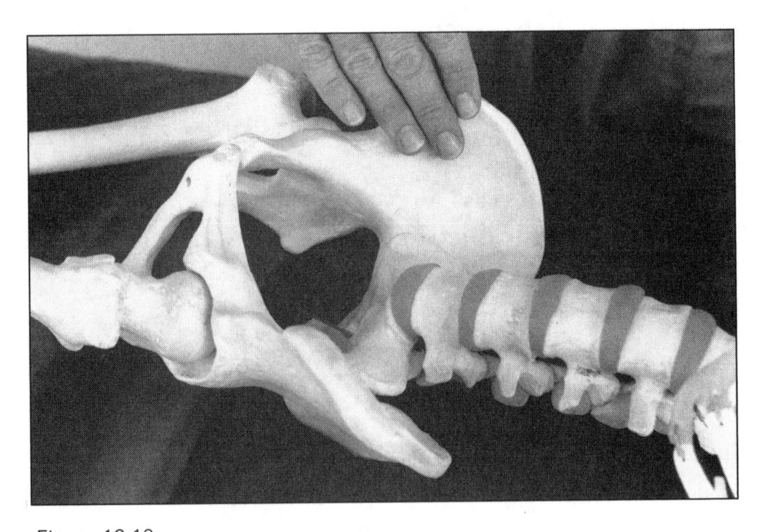

Figure 12.12

entry right along the edge of the right ASIS. Figure 12.11 also shows that the client has the legs extended. You will find that this technique can be much easier to accomplish if you have the knees flexed and rested together in the same way as pointed out in earlier techniques.

The starting point being on the medial edge of the ASIS, a slow gradual pressure is applied in a way that allows your fingers to curve around the edge of the iliac bone. It is as though you want your hands to follow the shape and contour of the bone rather than trying to get your fingers down toward the psoas, or even more medially, toward the spine. This area of the body is particularly sensitive in many people. It is here where five layers of fascia come together. It is here that the trunk and the pelvis meet the legs. So it is the confluence of many soft tissues, nervous, and circulatory processes in the body. Bear in mind that you should keep an eye on the client's face and breathing while you are doing this. Continue with your pressure until you meet a restriction barrier that can feel like a layer of tissue that is stuck or even hard. At this point, wait and hold, maintain your pressure, and ask the client to take a breath into your fingertips. As she exhales, instruct her to let go.

As an alternative, you can also have the client lift her tailbone up, and the reverse of that motion, press her tailbone into the table. Because there are at least five layers of fascia underneath your fingertips, you may very well feel as many as five releases. However, just one is enough, especially if the client is unfamiliar with this style of work in such a sensitive area. You will generally have more opportunities to come back to these issues around the psoas muscle. Another alternative for getting a release that is much more vigorous and can be used with a client accustomed to this style of work, is to have her lift the leg and foot one inch off the table. That is the leg or side that you are working on, and in this case, it is the right leg and right foot. When the leg is lifted in this manner, you will feel the tissue pull under your fingertips, and it is important to maintain your pressure, which at this point could be upward to 10 to 15 pounds and perhaps even more. Have the client extend her leg straight out very slowly, keeping the foot and leg about one inch above the table, and as soon as the leg is straight, have her flex it back up again. And as she is coming back up, release your pressure. It is important to remember here that the cecum also has a ligamentus attachment to the psoas muscle on the posterior aspect of the cecum. What this means is that problems such as chronic constipation, irritable bowel, and other nutritional/intestinal problems can reflex into the psoas and low back. This technique is recommended for those clients with low back, sacral, and leg problems, who have not been responding to other techniques you have employed.

The Work: Iliacus and Cecum

Client Position: Supine, with knees flexed, use strap if necessary

1. Place fingertips right along the medial aspect of the right ASIS.
2. Gradually apply enough pressure, so your fingers begin to curve around the edge of the iliac bone.
3. Just follow the contour of the bone.
4. Find restrictions, wait, hold, maintain pressure, and wait for softening.
5. While waiting, have the client breathe into your fingertips.
6. As she exhales, instruct her to let go.

Iliacus and Sigmoid Colon

These techniques may seem like the same technique for the iliacus and cecum; however, that is not the case. The structure of the sigmoid colon is very different than that of the cecum. The therapist's fingertips in Figure 12.13 are using a point of entry on the left hand side of the body that is just medial to the ASIS. The sigmoid colon

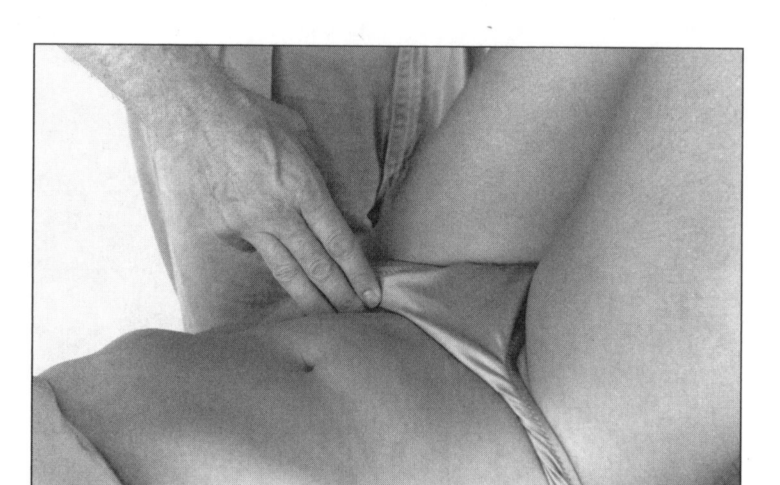

Figure 12.13

is near the end of the large intestine, and in many anatomy books, appears not unlike the drainpipe under every sink in your house. It has a big s-shaped curve and bends as it comes along the edge of the illiacus muscle in the iliac fossa. The sigmoid colon has a specialized fascia called the sigmoid mesacolon. This sigmoid mesacolon attaches the entire sigmoid to the illiacus and not the psoas.

The technique is done with your fingers pointed at an angle more toward the pelvis floor than the description on the preceding pages of the cecum release. This angle is important because of the deeper position that the sigmoid has in the floor of the pelvis. The technique in its application is at this point essentially the same as before, the client with her knees flexed, will lift her foot and leg up off the table and extend them. Alternately you can just go layer by layer and have her move her tailbone occasionally. Figure 12.14 shows a variation that can be done on both sides, and that is with your thumbs or fingertips. In this case, use your thumb because it is the easiest tool with the angle you are working at. Allow your thumb to sink into the abdomen right next or just medial to the ASIS until you feel the first restriction barrier. Then, scoop and lift

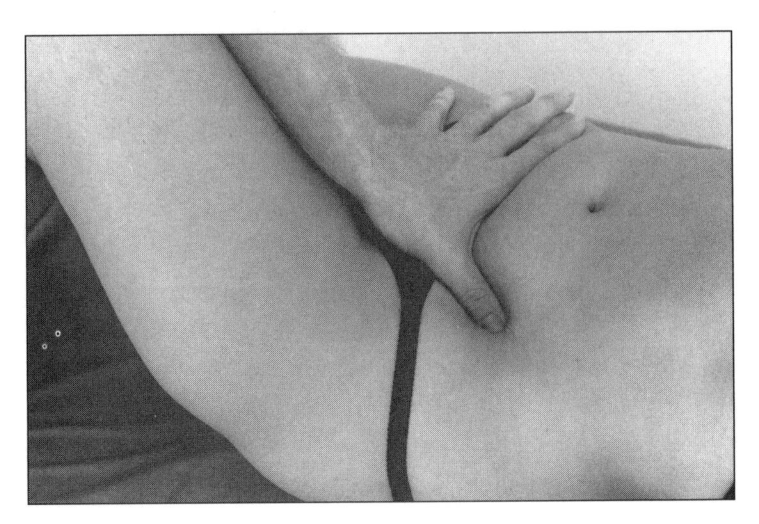

Figure 12.14

the tissue in small segments of an inch or two in length on a line going from the ASIS to the umbilicus.

Employ the same motion as before, tailbone up, tailbone down. Do this on both sides, and you will find it will have a dramatic effect, especially with those clients that have had surgery in the lower abdomen and pelvis. Those surgeries would include appendectomies, C-Sections, laparoscopies, hysterectomies, and so on. When you apply this technique to the right side around the cecum, it will also have a beneficial effect in toning the ileocecal valve. These fascia have continuity with the fascia of the pelvis floor and adductor. Generally speaking, when you work the adductors, you also work the iliopsoas. Then you do these two; finish the work in the lumbar fascia. They form an important trilogy of postural support fascia.

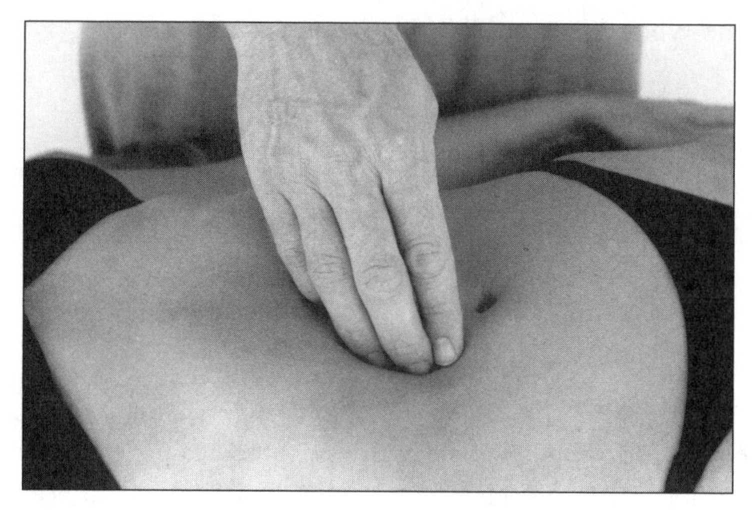

Figure 12.15

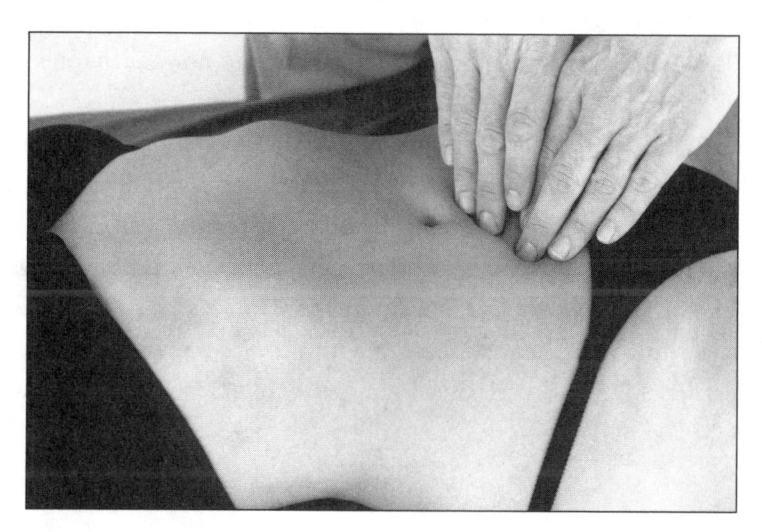

Figure 12.16

The Work: Iliacus and Sigmoid Colon

Client Position: Supine, with knees flexed, use strap if necessary

1. Using thumb or fingers, enter on the left side.
2. The vector is toward the pelvic floor, medial to the ASIS.

Root of the Mesentery and Palpation of the Duodenum

Figure 12.15 shows the therapist palpating the duodenum that is between the large intestine and the umbilicus. It is just below the surface of the rectus abdominus. It feels like a small flexible tube. His fingers are approximately where the Sphincter of Oddi is located. Massage in small clockwise circles to normalize tone in this important sphincter.

Figure 12.16 shows the therapist's hands on a line from the duojejunal junction to the right ASIS (anterior superior iliac spine). Gently weave your way to the posterior abdominal wall, and you will feel the root of the mesentery. This fascial connection always shortens after any abdominal surgery and needs to be released. Have the client bring her legs up with the knees resting together (feet spread) in order to put slack into the abdomen. Go slowly and avoid compressing the aorta.

SECTION 3

Commentaries

CHAPTER 13

The Structural Integration Model of Ida P. Rolf, Ph.D., by Michael J. Shea, Ph.D.

> *Part of a Rolfer's strategy consists in recognizing that the plasticity of the body has to do with the chemistry of that system of the body that creates and maintains structure—the myofascial system. Realize that this system derives from the mesoderm. Only this system do we manipulate directly, but by virtue of this system we can change the functioning of the entire body. We can change the verticality of the body. So that in this chemical elasticity of the myofascia you have a tool to effect lasting change. In addition, you have the segmentation of the body, which makes the tool usable. Why in heaven's name somebody down through these thousands of years didn't see this long before and use it, I'll never know.*
> (Rolf, 1978)

Ida P. Rolf, Ph.D. spent most of her adult life working on a model that involved organizing and integrating the soft tissue system of the body. This model has been called structural integration as well as Rolfing, since it became a formal system of training in the 1960s. The terms Rolfing, myofascial release, structural integration, deep tissue work, and the work of Ida P. Rolf are used interchangeably throughout this article. They derive from the same set of principles. The formulation of her ideas into a system of bodywork began much earlier in the teens and early 1920s.

Her original influences came from several disciplines, especially biochemistry, homeopathy, yoga, and osteopathy. Her doctoral work in biochemistry led her to understand the unique and complex properties of the fascial system. From her study of biochemistry and her work in the field of biochemistry at the Rockerfeller Institute in New York as well as her initial experiences of doing hands-on manipulation in the 1930s, she realized that the body is a plastic medium. This principle was a dramatic departure from the mechanistic approaches to orthopedics, and the fundamental medical understanding of the structure of the human body. This primary principle has gone through a maze of research down to the quantum level. This now includes an understanding of not only its plasticity, but also the electrical, chemical, and electromagnetic components of the fascial system.

The soft tissue of the body consists of muscles and its covering, the fascia. This soft tissue is also called the myofascia. Through all of the exhaustive research this principle still remains true: the body is a plastic medium. This notion is supported not only by biochemistry but also by the disciplines of quantum physics and psychology. The body as a plastic medium is a principle that quite simply demonstrates that thoughts and emotions shape the body, and the body shapes your emotional life (Pert, 1997). In terms of the work of Ida P. Rolf, this psychophysical principle forms a contemporary corollary to her foundation principle of structural integration that the body is a plastic medium. Add that the body is a fluid medium that may help understand what she was saying.

The homeopathic principle of like treats like influenced Ida Rolf in a number of ways. The first of these was the strategy of disease treatment: any treatment of a disease or illness process in the body should proceed layer by layer from outside to inside as though the pathology were an onion that needed to shed its skin one step at a time. Embryologically, a human organism develops as a whole, and thus must always be treated as a whole. Once a child is born and stands upright, his or her development then becomes bidirectional. The earth develops us from bottom to top, and society develops us from front to back. Ida Rolf developed a foundation strategy in her work that insisted that the superficial fascia of the body be organized and integrated prior to entering into the deep fascia of the body. It related to her perception that body problems needed direct input at the level that they entered the body. In other words, when a person sustains a high velocity impact trauma like a car accident, sometimes it is necessary to work the tissue deeply to match the strength of the injury.

The notion of like treats like and amplification gave rise to structural integration embodying the Christian metaphor of no pain no gain. This metaphor came from the sixth-century Christian scholar Ignatius of Antioch, and sees the life of the body as one of struggle and pain. The body is viewed as unhealthy, sinful, and the source of many potential evils; therefore, it should be vilified, torn down, or put through painful tests for its salvation. Then along comes Ida P. Rolf and her approach to body therapy: take the tissue into its anatomically correct position by force and ask for movement. The amount of force used may be great. In the early development of structural integration, the amount of pressure that was used could also be sustained for a whole hour, whereas now the deep pressure may only be a fraction of an hour. You could always count on a Rolfer to go deep into the body better than anyone else in the 1960s and 1970s.

This early sustained depth of touch elevated the work of Ida Rolf from a mere association with the Christian metaphor of no pain no gain into a type of mythology. When Burt Reynolds went to see Ida Pelf and got Pelfed in his movie "Semi Tough," Rolfing became elevated to a myth and synonymous with no pain no gain. It highlighted a systematic unconscious body of information about the nature of pain with which culture is fascinated. The belief of the culture is that by undergoing pain and trial you can be saved, and in this case, it is your body that needs salvation by the hands of a Rolfer. However, what one ultimately discovers by getting Rolfed is an awareness of how one holds onto his or her body and mind. That is the source of the pain. It comes from the inside. Even the thoughts one has about his or her body are in the body, and they may cause or exacerbate the pain. The sensation of being Rolfed is often misinterpreted as pain. This pain metaphor is one that the Rolf Institute and offshoot schools have been attempting to confront for the last two decades. It will always exist as part of the shadow side of doing deep tissue work like Rolfing. It goes with the territory. The inside of the body is a mystery, and those who journey there are often elevated to the status of a cult figure. Formerly only priests and physicians were allowed to know the inside of a body.

Ida Rolf borrowed a yogic principle and added it to her concept of structural integration: length in the joint spaces of the body promotes physical well-being. This principle gets translated into a strategy of tissue interaction while practicing structural integration. Yoga in general is a terrific support for a Rolfed body. A yoga practice clearly assists anyone who has undergone the Rolfing process. I know this to be true for my own body. When I received my original ten sessions of Rolfing back in the mid 1970s, it had very little effect at the time. I hardly felt the effect of the Rolfing work physically or emotionally. This was for several reasons. I was jogging three to five miles a day and practicing full contact karate regularly. However, several years later after I had taken up a regular yoga practice and stopped karate, I was in a class with my yoga teacher, and at the end of the class, I felt all ten sessions of my original Rolfing emerge in my body in a way I could utilize and integrate it into my current life experience. Somehow that yoga class evoked my original Rolfing sessions. That one yoga class and the body memories it brought up became a peak experience for me and one that I will never forget. Rolfing creates a body memory that is lasting and accessible long after the initial work.

Ida Rolf also incorporated the osteopathic principle of the inseparability of structure and function of the human body. For the early osteopaths as well as Ida Rolf, working on structure to affect function was foundational to any subsequent understanding of human structure and functioning. Although she claimed to not indulge much in the psychological interface with her work, the work she started has evolved into a finer understanding of the role that psychology plays in the shape and form of the human body. Working on structure affects function at every level. Some levels of structure are affected immediately, whereas other functional aspects of the body are affected more slowly and over a longer period of time, such as the nervous, immune, lymphatic, and cardiovascular systems. When you work directly on one system of the body as Rolfing does, it indirectly affects all the other systems of the body. This was also her way of getting around scientific reductionism and the roots of Cartesian duality or the mind/body split. She took her argument of the inseparability of mind and body into the physical domain of the structure and function of the human body. She always said that was because it was all you could get your hands on. Dr. Rolf's work focuses on the fascia of the body. This primary focus with the fascial system derives from osteopathy as well.

One of the main foundation principles that Ida Rolf developed was her notion that optimal function of the human body occurs when the structure of the body is aligned around a central vertical axis. Therefore, the goal of the work is to achieve this alignment within ten sessions. This principle has evolved over the years into establishing a more balanced relationship between external compressional forces, like gravity and accidents, and internal expansive forces in a dynamic, balanced, reciprocal tension. These balanced internal forces include biokinetic influences of fluid pressure against membrane and biodynamic forces of breathing, heart pumping, cranial rhythm, and so on. These forces are seen in action potentials that are generated by the DNA in a cell nucleus, and move out to the cell membrane and through it via complex bioelectric and biochemical reactions particularly in the endothelium of distressed tissue from an inflammatory diet.

The central vertical axis is a theoretic line of balance between buoyancy and gravity that is constantly shifting in a living moving body. The traditional style of Rolfing was very demanding around placement of the central vertical axis in alignment with the front of the spine. That fixed line, so to speak is no longer tenable in the process of organizing and integrating a body. There are numerous sociocultural relationships constantly influencing the shape of the body (e.g., family, friends, school, etc.) as well as internal subjective relationships between the various systems of the body and numerous mind/body variables (Pincus & Callahan, 1995). Balance is the key here, not symmetry. Humans are not designed embryologically to grow symmetrically (Blechschmidt & Gasser, 2012). Balance is a readiness to respond to random and fixed stimuli and implies flexibility. Balance is a state of equilibrium or equipoise between two parts that may in fact be in conflict such as the lift of buoyancy in the sum of all the fluids in the body and the downward drag of gravity on the fascia. Body equilibrium includes the relationship between the various parts of the body and the external environment that is constantly changing. Change process in the body is crucial to the work of Ida P. Rolf, Ph.D.

This notion of relationship is a foundational principle in Rolfing. To Ida Rolf, relationship was the key to her method of structural integration. She stressed the importance of seeing relationships in the fascial system through developing clear observation skills and the importance of building relationships in the body with her work. "Can you see relationship?" was the constant question that Ida Rolf asked her students when looking at someone's body. The various structural parts of the body are all related via the fascial system. She urged her students to see how a twisted ankle caused an entire chain of compensation up the leg into the back, girdles, and so on. It was not good enough to work on a sprained ankle without relating it to the rest of the body.

In order to see relationship as Ida Rolf exhorted her students, it is no longer possible to bodily exist in a realm of objective symmetry. The subjective first-person experience of the therapist feeling and perceiving his or her body and an in-depth understanding of the neuroscience of interpersonal neurobiology is included. Perhaps it is correct to say that relationship is everything. It was not possible in the early stages in learning to Rolf to include an expanded curriculum with the new science of interpersonal neurobiology. It was enough to learn the complex global strategies of intervention that Rolfing employs. Now, however, as culture moves into a more connected understanding of life, it is imperative that everyone, both clients and therapists, study the new science of interpersonal neurobiology (Siegel, 1999).

Mindfulness is the emerging field that is being integrated with the manual therapeutic arts. Mindfulness describes the conscious experience of inhabiting a living body and refers to the ongoing process of embodiment without judgment or interpretation. The perceptions of the therapist are linked to his or her sensate experience. This is how to try to educate clients, that is, to continually link feelings, emotions, and perceptions to sensations arising in the body with mindfulness. The ability to identify sensation mindfully is curative by itself. Rolfing is a mindful art because it seeks to educate the client regarding sensory experience around an internal vertical axis and within the field of gravity. At the same time, to move within the currents and fluid dynamics of all living systems requires an awareness of the inside of the body and its fluid sensuality and spontaneous movement. Sensory perception is a collaborative event when a therapist works with a client. The client is sensing the therapist as much as the therapist is sensing the client. This is resonance and is at the heart of mindfulness. Thus the healing or curative effect of Rolfing is once again associated with mindfulness of the relationship. This time it is a relationship between the therapist's sensory perceptions and the client's sensory perceptions.

The evolution of Ida Rolf's work has borrowed the principle of holism from humanistic psychology (Maslow, 1971) and the principle of emergence from the new biology (Harman, 1995). The concept of holism includes a principle that body and mind are indivisible, which sounds very similar to the idea of the inseparability of structure and function. Mind and body are separate but equal as well as being indivisible. The conscious ability to hold this ambiguity is a mark of a self-actualized person according to Maslow. It is not so much that Maslow meant holding the mind/body ambiguity, but rather ambiguity in general of which existential meaning-making, mind/body complex is but one of many ambiguities or paradoxes that one must come to grips with in this life. The complexity of mind/body interactions is a central tenet of Ida Rolf's work and includes evoking self-regulation from the body. Self-regulation is the felt sense of an internal ability to lower states of autonomic activation. Self-regulation is a function of an interconnected brain and heart and fluid body that is held mindfully. It builds resilience (Davidson & Begley, 2012). There is a life principle that is critical to structural integration and may be forgotten by the client. The process of Rolfing has the ability to wake up this life principle or intelligence of self-regulation and resilience.

Rolfing creates a set of circumstances, sometimes referred to as space in the client's body for the emergence of fluid movement to occur. In this context, the challenge to anyone practicing Rolfing (or any manual therapeutic art) is to have stereoscopic vision. On the one hand, hypothesizing that balance around a central vertical axis is what a body wants for its well-being, and on the other hand, one must also allow for creative emergence of fluidity to occur in whatever shape and form it wants to and not interfere with its chosen path, but rather offer what emerges the possibility of physical structural integration (Conrad, 2007). The whole is held in the vision and particulars. Fluid fascial bodies are designed for learning. Rolfing can facilitate this biological law. This is the nature of having a body that is predominantly made of biological water, as it is now known that 99 percent of the molecules in the body are water molecules (Pollack, 2013). "A Rolfer must be able to be comfortable with phenomena that are always shifting, always moving" (Rolf, 1978, p. 53).

> *Start at the outside and work in. Most manipulative therapies start at the inside, at what they say is the "cause." Maybe it is the cause; I don't care if it is. But I say you can't start there. You've got to start where you can unwind the trouble.*
> (Rolf, 1978, p. 153)

CHAPTER 14

The Expression of the Autonomic Nervous System

Traditionally, the autonomic nervous system (ANS) is viewed as a system composed of two antagonists: the sympathetic nervous system and the parasympathetic nervous system. The sympathetic nervous system is the part that elicits fight-or-flight responses. However, the current paradigm about these two parts of the autonomic nervous system is that they are not antagonistic systems, but rather that the sympathetic nervous system is primarily a mediator between the neuromuscular system and the visceral system (Korr, 1979). All soft tissue has sympathetic innervation. There is virtually no parasympathetic innervation of soft tissue. All of the cardiovascular system, every blood capillary in the body, has a sympathetic nerve attached to it. Therefore, the sympathetic nervous system regulates the vasomotor system. The rate and flow of the blood through the body is controlled by the sympathetic nervous system. The vagus nerve, which represents 75 percent of the parasympathetic system, has some control over the heart and visceral system. Everything else is sympathetic, throughout the whole body. The contraction/dilation of the blood vessels (vasomotor) is accomplished via the sympathetic nervous system.

The parasympathetic part helps regulate the visceral system (which is all of the organs—the digestive apparatus) and forms a link to the enteric nervous system for cross-talk to the central nervous system (Camilleri, 1993). The main part of the parasympathetic system is the vagus nerve, and in the pelvis it is the sacrococcygeal plexus. The parasympathetic system is called the cranial-sacral system, and the sympathetic system is called the thoracolumbar system. This represents where the nerve roots originate respectively.

There is a tuning process between the sympathetic nervous system (neuromuscular system and cardiovascular systems) and the visceral system (parasympathetic nervous system). The neuromuscular system is the largest consumer of energy in the body. It uses more oxygen and produces more heat and waste products more rapidly than any other part of the body. This requires the sympathetic nervous system to modulate and tune visceral functioning to respond to the needs of the neuromuscular system (Gellhorn, 1960). Thus, it is considered to be a primary system. The neuromuscular system in this paradigm is considered to be primary because it is the biggest consumer of energy in the whole system. The viscera contain their own inertia and have a smaller influence on the spinal cord and brain (Foreman, 1989). The viscera and enteric system, which are the neurons in the alimentary canal, keep digesting food and producing amino acids and fatty acids and fuel for metabolism. When one exercises improperly or lives with a lot of stress and anxiety, it tightens the soft tissue. Then the visceral system will begin to decrease activity because of the energy shift into the soft tissue. Over time, this imbalance becomes the general adaptive response (Selye, 1976). Soft tissue dysfunction and visceral problems (ulcers, constipation, irritable bowel syndrome, diarrhea, etc.) become prominent. Continued habituation becomes adaptive and compromises the immune system, heart, and brain (Arnason, 1993). Habituation is the first stage of stress responses in the body until the nervous system charges and adapts to elevated levels of charge and stimulation known as stress.

The central nervous system provides the basic wiring for muscular activity. Research has shown that the sympathetic innervation in the soft tissue augments muscle energy (Korr, 1979). The body receives a 20 percent boost in muscle energy activity by stimulating the sympathetic fibers in the soft tissue. This is in addition to the capacity of the central nervous system afferents. Muscle tissue contains both types of nervous innervation, sympathetic and somatic. This gives the soft tissue system of the body tremendous adaptive potential when under threat, performing, and so on. Under emotional stress, the energy in the sympathetic system increases. One has heard all the stories about people who lift cars up off kids who have been hit, and other dramatic feats of strength. It is also referred to as second wind in sports—it is really important information for myofascial release. Any time you lay your hands on somebody, you can begin affecting sympathetic tone. The current culture breeds very high sympathetic tone, which goes hand-in-hand with having to run five yellow lights (and maybe a couple of red ones) on the way to work every morning, while consuming three cups of coffee and having an argument with your wife on the car phone, and facing an angry boss. The same response that primitive people had to a sabertooth tiger attack is the same response as when a person today almost gets hit by a car. The nervous system initiates the same response as the primitive man's. However, today a person cranks up his or her nervous system far more often than the primitive man did, and then keep it up with poor diet, lifestyle, and so on. It gets stuck on this high. It was not designed for this (Levine, 1986). The natural response is not completed. This is extremely relevant in the myofascial release concept because this incomplete response is found in the connective tissue.

It is not unusual at all during myofascial release to begin seeing a tone shift within 5, 10, 15 minutes. What is normally looked for is lower tone. Those clients who feel dizzy, who start to sweat (sudomotor response), or whose whole body flushes and shakes from myofascial release, are demonstrating a rapid tone shift in the entire sympathetic nervous system. Accumulated stress, anxiety, and neurological reflex activity have a direct relationship to the physical trauma with which is being worked. The body collects not only on the trauma that has occurred, but also on the general adaptive response (Willard & Patterson, 1992). If perspectives are broadened just a little bit, one can begin to see tone shifts and look for them in the skin color, sweating, emotional responses, shaking, and so on. When one starts doing fascial manipulation, one must keep his or her eyes open and scan the body. With any kind of bodywork, one can begin to observe sympathetic tone shift or discharge phenomena. It makes the work a whole lot easier.

Some of the preverbal signals that the body gives off have been mentioned. The terms used are sympathetic tone shift or discharge phenomena. What these terms mean is that high sympathetic tone will begin to shift the moment you begin applying manual therapy. This is a bold statement but, all manual therapy causes the autonomic nervous system to shift. This autonomic expression happens in a wide variety of ways. For example, fasciculation activity: a client's leg begins trembling or his or her arm or shoulder starts to shake. It is not unusual at all. Clients need permission for these responses to occur. Clients start shaking almost uncontrollably or trembling. Trembling, shaking, jerking, skin color changes, sweating, clamminess, laughing, crying; these are autonomic discharge patterns (Levine, 1992). Have you ever noticed how sometimes in the middle of a treatment somebody will begin talking a lot? That is another sign of sympathetic discharge. The verbal system becomes activated. This also applies to crying. How many people have had a client or a patient cry with them? This is sympathetic discharge. The hypothalamus coregulates the autonomic nervous system. It is the end structure in the limbic system or mid-brain. The emotions interface with the body via the limbic system (LeDoux, 1993). Emotions form an interface with the hypothalamus (reaction), hippocampus (memory), and especially the amygdala (emotion)—all limbic structures. These three structures are right next to each other (Morgane, 1992). Recent research (Pert, 1995) indicates that neurotransmitters regulate moon and emotions. The majority of receptor sites for these transmitters are in the amygdala hippocampus and hypothalamus.

What are emotions? What is anger? In the spectrum of anger, there is rage and hatred. What is a lesser variation of anger? Disgust. Others are aggression and irritation. It is called gauze-like irritation—the web of irritation felt every now and then. This irritation is actually quite healthy and relates to mindfulness and awareness of the environment. Very often the environment is giving reminders by way of an irritating quality to pay attention and become more aware of what's going on within you and outside of you. The bodies shape around the emotions (Reich, 1997). When you hold onto your emotions for awhile, the hypothalamus begins to regulate the neuromuscular desire to swing at your boss, or shake a fist at the driver who almost hit you. You hold onto what happens to you in the soft tissue and fascia. Most cervical whiplash injuries are accompanied by fear, anxiety, and high sympathetic tone. Whiplash patients were usually on their way from or to an emotionally charged situation. It is important to ask the client where they were coming from or going to. Then there are those with multiple motor vehicle accidents (MVAs). Ask the client what he or she has learned from all the accidents. What is the message? Has he or she gotten the message? There is an important psychological interface with stress, illness, and soft tissue problems that cannot be ignored (Booth & Ashbridge, 1993; Cunningham, 1955; Foss, 1994; Squotas-Emch, Glaser, & Kiecolt-Glaser, 1992).

To differentiate between a release and a discharge, the autonomic system discharges, the soft tissue system releases; it is a continuum or cycle. When the energy of a soft tissue release shunts into the autonomic nervous system, it will do that because this is all predicated on the bioelectrical activity and bioenergetic level within the tissue that triggers a discharge. This is defining a discharge as a much broader-based, whole-system event. A release is a more regional situation in the soft tissue. Discharge is systemic. It is a larger whole-system or multisystem event. The fascial system releases down in a leg. The respiratory system begins to constrict and hold or hyperventilate, which is parasympathetic. Tears begin to form in the eyes. Sympathetic tone is shifting. This is a multisystems event. The central nervous system and the autonomic nervous system may desynchronize for several minutes. This can be crying or having a catharsis, genuine unwinding, or even dissociation. This is discharge. The body is facilitating this response and helping to guide it to resolution. The skill of the therapist is important. The discharge needs to be acknowledged and supported. You may suspend your treatment plan and shift gears into tracking the autonomic nervous system.

The key is going slowly, backing off, and watching people breathe to allow an integration to occur in the nervous system. Integration refers to the adaptability of the brain or body to a higher level of functioning. It implies the nervous system seeking wholeness and healing from its fragmentation. Integration implies that the discharge process is enhancing organismic functioning. Integration is a function of time. The nervous system takes more time to integrate than soft tissue does to release. This integration may not complete itself for hours or days after it is initiated by the work. Integration does not complete itself while the client is in the office. Allow the leg, hip, or spine that has become orthopedically involved to release, then allow the client to move through discharge and then integrate through the whole nervous system and body. It is a permission that you are giving the client. It requires patience, vision, and a soft touch on your part.

With any particular trauma in a person's life, there are always some related events occurring psychologically and physically. Holistic, humanistic models postulate that mind and body are inseparable (Cassidy, 1994; Johnson, 1983, 1994). But practitioners are not attempting to be psychotherapists at all. If you can just open your eyes and observe tone shifts happening as releases and then discharges; give people verbal permission; and keep them breathing into the pain (because that is what practitioners are really concerned about here—how to bring order and utilize and integrate discharge phenomena), you will do your patients and clients a great service. What you often miss in terms of observation skills is scanning the whole body when the client walks in for his or her appointment and all the nonstructural cues just mentioned. Practitioners have all gotten good at symmetrical/structural observation in standing. Now I suggest that you can begin to observe the autonomic nervous system, which is not symmetrical. The brain and spinal cord map out reflex activity for pain (nociception), emotion, sensation, feeling, thoughts, and so on, to the body (Willard & Patterson, 1992). It is unique to the individual, observable and very workable. The face, jaw, eyes, neck, trunk, breathing, extremities, and pelvis are the areas where the major autonomic plexi are located. Autonomic activation and discharge are highly observable in these areas.

As the sympathetic nervous system tone drops, parasympathetic tone rises or rebounds (Gellhorn, 1957). There are specific areas of the body, particularly the lumbar fasciae and the cervical fasciae, that when manipulated, will raise vagal tone (Cottingham, Porges, & Lyon, 1988; Cottingham, Porges, & Richmond, 1988). Cranial-sacral work also raises vagal tone. As mentioned earlier, these areas of the body contain the integrative fascias—all the paraspinal fascias. These fascias are integrative because you work on them at the end of every session. It puts the whole session together by organizing the paraspinal fascias toward the midline. Sometimes this vagal parasympathetic shift feels like nausea or a slight headache, or the spine will arch into extension. These are transient sensations. Sometimes the sensation associated with these autonomic shifts are pleasurable, and clients could be reminded of this and asked to smile. The face is a parasympathetic organ, and smiling activates the parasympathetic system (Ruskin, 1979).

The breath has such a big impact because systemically, by working with the breath along with sympathetic discharge, there is a reeducation and reintegration that occurs very deep inside a person. Most people do not know how to breathe into pain. Culture is oriented around breath-holding—a fixation on either exhalation or inhalation. The startle-reflex mechanism in the respiratory diaphragm becomes fixated. It is as though people are holding their breath waiting for all these feelings to go away and to leave them alone. There is a blockage, or a lack of synchronization between sympathetic discharge, emotional arousal, and the way that emotions are experienced in the body. Think about your experience. Philosophers and scientists have been arguing for a long time about the actual experience of emotion (Solomon, 1993). But one can be quite pragmatic and recognize that when he or she feels excitement, anger, passion, sadness, guilt, and so on, the person does feel it in the body. You might remember having the experience of being angry and having sensations rushing through your arms and legs and chest, or noting that sadness has a definite location in the upper thoracic area, maybe the chest. By working with the client's breath, you actually can reconnect or synchronize the body and mind during myofascial release, or any bodywork for that matter. It does not have to be cathartic or something wild.

The clinical applications are quite amazing. Think if you could affect the whole body without using hot packs or cold packs or ultrasound. Think if you had a way of supporting vasodilation systemically, if you had a way of supporting metabolic waste removal systemically, wouldn't you want to do that? If you move slowly into the tissue, if you are not looking at it as simply a mechanical procedure, you then have the opportunity to reduce sympathetic dominance. Systemic vasodilation is important, and systemic waste removal is also important, because where you have increased blood flow, you are going to decrease nerve irritation. Also, with the decrease in sympathetic tone, you have more blood shunting into the viscera. There is such a large problem with ulcers and a host of related digestive disorders. It is a sign of high sympathetic dominance and the general adaptive response. An increase in systemic waste removal, vasodilation, and relaxation in the soft tissue are going to help your work because what you are intending is to facilitate a healing response in the body and let the body take over its own healing. The breath influences so much physiology systemically. The body wants to balance itself. Part of the physiology of stress is that the higher the percentage of carbon dioxide in the blood, the more acidic the blood becomes, and therefore, the greater the tendency on an intercellular level for hypoxia. This strangles the body's healing response. As you encourage slow, full, purposeful breathing, you are flooding the body with oxygen. The experience of tetany that some of you might see in doing this work is simply the body's transition state out of one homeostatic level to another. When a client goes into tetany, encourage relaxation with the breath, and massage the client's arms and face to relieve the cramping. Tetany occurs because hyperventilation causes the calcium ion pump to shunt calcium out of the muscle. This causes cramping in the arms and face in particular, along with a numbing sensation in the lips. The client will also begin to curl up into fetal position and hyperflex his or her wrists, elbows, and arms.

The first treatment goal is always to promote flexibility in the autonomic nervous system by reducing sympathetic adaptation and inputting to the parasympathetic areas of the body. Can you be flexible enough to shift your goals in the middle of a treatment? When you see discharge beginning, you might say, "Oh, this is obviously a sympathetic tone drop, crying, shaking, whatever," and shift your approach away from the tissue and your goals for the session at that point. The strategy in a discharge is to organize the bioenergy and movement of the discharge up and down the axial midline of the body. Or if the middle is bound up, then move the discharge out to the extremities. Then integrate that discharge into their central nervous system and throughout their body? Change your goals and intervention strategies to accommodate any state change in the client. Follow their process as they switch body systems. If they are sympathetically dominant at the beginning of the treatment and then become parasympathetic dominant, you cannot continue the same level of touch. Your touch must change. Sometimes that means cranial work, other times it means gently holding the client's diaphragm or massage or movement work or nothing at all. Let go of always doing something to the client. Develop or cultivate a simple presence, keep your eyes open, and be available to support the client.

Coupled with the capability to have a flexible approach in the treatment is the ability to move from an area of specificity to a more global view. You can step back and look at the whole person. You can encourage emotional integration through hands-on contact. Your caring can be expressed through your hands, and you can encourage integration by reminding or educating your patients to relax through their breath. It is very simple. You can encourage clients to give feedback about the pressure used. It does not involve any analysis, and you begin to respect the person's ability to integrate on their own. You can be there as a facilitator and educator, not just a technician. That is a very powerful clue for patients, just to encourage breathing and verbal feedback. What you are addressing here is trust that develops through intimacy. Breathing is very intimate. In society, intimacy is immediately paired with sexuality, and that is a big mistake because it denies a majority of intimate contact that people have and do not notice. There is the intimacy of one's own gentleness. That is really the focus in the work—one's own gentleness. You are not interested in just teaching slick techniques.

There are intelligent ways to interface with autonomic arousal. If you see someone's leg begin to shake, you may ask, "Can you let the shaking into your pelvis?" Whenever there is a body part shaking, in terms of facilitating whole body integration, just see where the shaking is not happening, and ask if a person could go inside and allow that shaking to happen at the next segment higher or lower.

Move segment by segment. This might feel risky if you have not worked with these responses before. But you will be able to help that person more deeply. You are helping reconnect their whole body. The central nervous system loves that. It loves feeling the whole body rather than the fragmentation resulting from trauma. Many people experience themselves as fragmented without a sense of a whole. As a manual therapist, you can facilitate psychological integration. You are entering into a person's physical reality with empathy and an innate desire to help a person feel whole. That is big magic in indigenous cultures.

When you see discharge happening, breathing in the trunk and abdomen tends to become restricted. You can encourage relaxation in the abdomen and diaphragm verbally or just by placing your hand there. The thoracic outlet and the neck begin to tighten and flex during discharge. Perhaps you have seen that. You can encourage easing the neck by placing your hand under the neck or spine and gently lifting the spine into extension until you feel relaxation. This encourages the parasympathetic nervous system to open. This supports the charge to go through the body. An increase in parasympathetic tone is occurring when the body begins to go through a whip-like motion up and down the spine. Every now and then clients will get a sudden jerk in the body and arch the spine. This is the parasympathetic tone, the vagal tone is pushing right through because it has an opportunity to do so. This is to be supported because that tone shift will even out after a couple of minutes, perhaps as much as 15 or 20 minutes. Autonomic nervous system discharge patterns move back and forth from sympathetic to parasympathetic.

The task is to coach the breathing and to facilitate relaxation in the tight parts. You will see people trying to hold and constrict. Encourage them to let go of the holding in that area. If a client cannot let go, encourage getting in touch with the tight parts, getting to know them, as they have served a useful purpose. You do not want to ask a client to give up the fight without his or her permission. Some of you only have 20 minutes behind your curtains with people, and if this starts in the 15th minute, you have got 5 minutes. You have to shut it down, and you have work to do, but you also have a window of opportunity in future treatments to work with these responses. Any loss of short-term progress will be balanced by a greater gain in long-term effect coupled with improved client responsibility. This is quite simple and quite straightforward, although some of it looks a little strange from time to time.

During myofascial release treatments, pressure is applied to a specific layer of the connective tissue matrix. Factors of vector, duration, and movement of the patient's body can describe these maneuvers. In any case, the intended result of the work is to increase the mobility of the connective tissue. There are many clinical implications of this mobility, from improving local metabolic function to the potential for orthopedically realigning muscle groups and postural components. The fact that these results can occur from placing described pressure on connective tissue is a matter of clinical knowledge. Understanding how, anatomically, these changes can occur comes from the biochemical studies of piezoelectric effects in organic crystalline structures.

Piezo refers to any process involving pressure—in piezoelectronics, to produce changes in electrical fields.

At a molecular level, the tissues of the myofascial system are arranged as organic crystalline structures. As such, they have the capacity to generate and conduct electrical fields. The more hydrated the tissue, the better it performs its electrical duties. These duties include the ionic bonding and transfer of nutrients and wastes and the conducting of neural transmissions. Tissue under stress from injury, load, or lack of movement dehydrates, thereby decreasing the local electrical potential and interfering with metabolic functions.

The components of connective tissue are long, thin, flexible filaments of collagen surrounded by ground substance. The ground substance is composed of 30–40 percent glycosaminoglycans and 60–70 percent water. Together the glycosaminoglycans and water form a gel. This gel functions as a lubricant and to maintain space (known as critical fiber distance) between the collagen fibers. Any dehydration of the ground substance will decrease the free gliding of the collagen fibers. When critical fiber distance decreases, collagen fibers bond together to strengthen the fascial web in which muscles, bones, and organs live.

Applying pressure to any crystalline lattice increases its electrical potential, attracting water molecules, thus hydrating the area. This is the piezoelectric effect of manual connective tissue therapy. This hydration occurs rapidly in the ground substance. This is the first step in recovering mobility in the connective tissue.

In order for piezoelectric fields to be generated, proper vectors must be used. (A vector is a factor of both angle and force.) This is where the craft of myofascial release comes into play. Effective coordination of the appropriate pressure, angle, and duration of the maneuver can come only with sensitivity, training, and practice.

CHAPTER 15

Myofascial Release and the Psychosomatic Body

The psychology of myofascial release is asked about quite frequently. A specific psychology of fascial release is not known. However, it is known that collagen density (fascia) will shorten and thicken because of behaviorally mediated patterns of stress (Keleman, 1985). The rate of assembly of tight fascia exceeds the rate of removal. If you continue to posture the body a certain way (chest caved in, head forward or dropped, pelvis tucked, shoulders rounded, etc.) in response to negative and hostile feelings from yourself and others, you will surely build extra fascia to hold you in that posture. Thus your psychology is linked to your physiology (Reich, 1945).

It is also not unusual for an orthopedic injury to occur during an emotionally stressful time. A client had broken her arm in an automobile accident two years prior to visiting her therapist with a sore elbow. As her arm was worked on, she remembered that her brother had committed suicide three days before the auto accident. When she broke her arm, her cycle of grieving was cut short and delayed. She cried for over an hour while her therapist held her, then the pain in her arm slowly disappeared.

Always ask the clients what they were feeling at the time of their injury. The answers are surprising, especially with whiplash patients. There is this other body that individuals all carry around called the psychosomatic body. It is the body individuals think about (Am I too fat, too skinny...), obsess about (I'd love five more pounds on my shoulder girdle; I hate my thighs), or project onto (I wish my body had so-and-so's shape, if only I had her hair and complexion). Individuals have many thoughts that are inaccurate, unfair, or unrealistic about their bodies, all of which comprise the psychosomatic body. This body is also to be found in the fascia. The fascia is so remarkable that it will build just about any shape that one wants.

The principles of myofascial release try to discover who is really there behind all that tight fascia and high sympathetic tone and then to contact that person. It is possible to uncover a very healthy relationship with your body through the use of fascial manipulation—when it is properly applied. It is also possible to see this as you stand the client up and look at them nonstructurally. How does that person live in that body? What is that body trying to say? What part stands out, and what part do you avoid? The clients are obviously much more than an orthopedic injury.

With a slight shift in your perspective and technique, you can see another world and another body in the client that you may have guessed was there but could not quite put your finger on. It is also possible to deepen the relationship with the client by relating to your own feelings of inadequacy, doubt, and embarrassment—particularly around the work you are doing with clients. Psychologically, when you become aware of another, or in this case look at the client before, during, and after a session, three things are happening in your field of experience:

- Your eyes, hands, and other senses are drawn to certain anatomical parts.
- You miss or do not see certain other anatomy.
- You are repulsed or pushed away from other anatomy.

Then you add a conceptual overlay or metaphysical template on top of this experience. If you have been trained to be a good Rolfer or physical therapist, you will see lack of symmetry. If you are not good at working with knees, you will avoid them. However, mind is also a sense organ, so on some level, you may be thinking that this person is sexy and you want to sleep with him or her, so you are drawn to work the pelvis. Or, this person is big and strong and reminds you of your authoritarian father who physically abused you as a child, and you do a lot of back work because you can not face him. This can go on in your mind both consciously and unconsciously. Either way it will effect your behavior and work. The drive for clinical expertise in the field avoids the richness of the subjective information from where intuitive, creative, artistic, bodywork comes. You need to travel freely between both worlds. The data emerging from cognitive scientists is that one experiences before they know. Subjectivity precedes objectivity. Emotions precede lumbosacral dysfunction. Feelings about a client precede your clinical understanding of his or her physical dysfunction. Maslow said that one cannot know the whole. Experientially, you get little pieces of data from time to time about the client in your own psyche that you need to amplify to achieve art in your work, and art lies within the realm of subtleties and subjectivity.

Direct fascial manipulation accesses the subjective experience of a person's self. Individuals all have a rich inner life of thoughts, feelings, and emotions that contribute to the sense of self and body image. This sense of self and body image is impacted with manual therapy. This is the arena where a more genuine healing can occur. Often people say, "Boy, I'm finally feeling myself again and I didn't even know I was gone," or "I'm feeling life in that area that I haven't felt for ages."

The process of disease and illness often starts with self-alienation. It is a slow process of distancing from the self and the body, from the thought process and feelings, and then from others. It occurs simultaneously in the fascial system as well. Illness permeates both the mind and the body, and the fascia offers a possible link between the two. You can most certainly get your hands on it, as Ida Rolf said. Stress, immune system deficiency, the fight or flight reflexes, anxiety, and depression all take their toll on the soft tissue system of the body.

A deep-seated innate tendency toward health and well-being permeates the mind and body all the time, too. So, you may ask yourself, when you look at clients, "Where is the health in this person, where is the trauma?" Myofascial release involves learning the use of direct techniques, the interrelationship of the fascia, with the autonomic nervous system and the breath, and finally, the psychology of client-therapist relationships.

When you work with an intention to manipulate the fascia, you are theoretically affecting the whole. However, it takes more than one session to effectively integrate and organize the fascia to a higher level of functioning, especially since the depth you are achieving under your hands is on the level of the periosteum and the subserous fasciae (pleura), and even the dura mater. So you are affecting very deep structures just by the intention to work the fascia. Intention is "that which precedes action," so it is the mental coordination of thoughts and energy directed through your hands into the client. Many clients may feel their whole body being affected by local fascial manipulation. The client's awareness of this comes from the soft tissue and the autonomic nervous system. The autonomic nervous system regulates emotions. The benefit to the client is known only to him or her in the fullness of his or her own time. Yes, you can measure improvements in range of motion and so forth, but the client remains fragmented if the emotional component is not resolved and integrated. You do this by slowing your touch down, taking breaks from inputting to the client, and letting him or her breathe. It is a simple flow.

In conclusion, you may be fooling yourself about wanting to cure clients or provide some rescue for them. Although cures are certainly wonderful and do happen, it is truly an art form just learning how to be with people here and now in a nonjudgmental, intimate way. This involves much more than bodywork or psychological techniques—rather it goes to the heart of being authentically human (Trungpa, 1980).

CHAPTER 16

The Psychology of Pain in Musculoskeletal Dysfunction

Getting to the roots of physical pain in clients often proves to be an elusive game of cat and mouse. Each reported symptom leads you off on another merry chase from one anatomical landmark to another. Every now and then you get lucky, and the pain disappears, but your luck runs out the next day when the patient calls to announce that it has returned with a fury. Nowadays, clients present complex physical problems; they have often seen numerous other health professionals and may feel hopelessness. This essay covers four types of psychological pain that are interrelated with the physical.

Aloneness

The first type of pain is the pain of aloneness. There is hardly anyone who does not feel alone from time to time. One can have a fight with a loved one and feel isolated with frustrations, not knowing whom to turn to and, in some cases, not wanting to turn to anyone at all. This feeling of aloneness is like a cocoon with an invisible, but nonetheless solid, wall between the person and others. One must come to grips with his or her feelings and self, and it is not unusual for this sense of aloneness to escalate into feelings of loneliness. When one feels lonely, one often changes his or her behavior to avoid this intensification process. An individual may act out, become compulsive, or hurt his or her body. Physical pain often leads to the pain of aloneness, and likewise, being alone can lead to physical hurt. The mind and body are connected. Illness leads to isolation. You can relate to the client's isolation if you recognize this as an experience you have in your own life.

Depression

Second, depression is a pain, as you know. It is much deeper and richer than being alone. Healthy depression can prompt a life review that allows one to look at his- or herself very clearly and sometimes more vividly. Depression, when it is uncomplicated, is normal. It is an opportunity to withdraw, break contact, and examine the circumstances, relationships, troubles, and states of mind and body that the recent (and not so recent) past has provided. Healthy depression is impermanent, although it may not seem like it at the time. It is also an excellent opportunity to change things one does not like, to muster up the courage to confront inner oppressors, to choose a different way. Acute and chronic physical pain leaves clients debilitated and often depressed. Depression allows them to examine other factors that may be involved with their physical discomfort that they have overlooked. It is a chance to go inside.

If you really examine your aloneness and depression, it feels warm, cozy, and even comfortable. It is part of the richness of your inner life, your secret life that you hide from others. Clinical depression is an unhealthy depression that persists for a long time and needs to be treated by a professional.

Hope and Fear

The third type of pain is the pain of hope and fear—the ups and downs of life. In adolescence this is called flip/flop; in adult jargon it is called manic depression or mood swings. You have seen how painful adolescence is (either in yourself or your children) when one minute they are seemingly on top of the world and the next moment their world has collapsed on top of them. As an adult, you have good days and bad days. You have good hours sometimes followed by bad hours, moments, and so on. A bad day starts when you spill your coffee on your pants driving to work. It starts to rain, and the defroster does not work, forcing you to use your hand (or your shirt sleeve) to clear the fog. The rain has caused you to be late for work, and when you arrive, you find you have forgotten an important set of notes you have been working on. You are steaming by now, so you have an extra cup of coffee to whip your nervous system into shape. The first five clients you call have their answering machines on or are not available. You open the newspaper and are confronted with the latest tragedy. Lunch does not help because you must wait in line, and they run out of the food you wanted, so you must settle for a greasy burger. You are up for a short while. Then your boss gives you a new deadline. And, what about getting the car fixed? It is endless and irritating, this up and down of your existence. That energy is painful. Clients often have a string of nagging physical insults that bring them to your office. When will the pain end? When will it be over? How often are you asked these questions? It gets more hopeful and then relapse, better, then relapse. Everyone has their ups and downs, so you resort to wishful thinking and fantasy to relieve the load. That creates another fall from grace as well. You daydream or become forgetful. You develop mindless practices or become addictive. Physical pain accelerates this process.

One psychology professor said that the best psychology was really exquisite social work. Underneath much of a client's dilemma is poor time management, lack of qualified babysitters, credit cards that are at maximum, addictive behaviors/relationships, and checkbooks that do not balance. Physical dysfunction is a natural harbinger of needed change. It is a wake up call that must be heeded. It offers us the potential for change.

Pain of Pain

The fourth type of pain is the pain of pain. Pain begets pain. One's awareness is drawn to one's pain. You focus on it and exacerbate it. You now know how some people get locked into chronic pain, how the nociceptive (pain) nerves change their morphology and stay stimulated even after the external pain stimulus is gone. The nervous system has an evolutionary demand to pay attention to pain, and you live in a day and age of constant stimulation. You have lost the ability to slow down and relax and your body suffers from this. Your psyche suffers from this. At every level your pain will bring more pain because of the plasticity of your nervous system and the ability of your psyche to plum the depths of your unconscious and allow more pain—the pain of pain to surface.

Clients often have a look of fear along with their physical problems. Fear is natural and normal. It can protect one from harm and is considered an instinctual drive rather than an emotion. Any physical illness will scare you. You may have a sore throat one day, and the next day be convinced that you have cancer. It is so refreshing to wake up on the fourth day and be all better and laugh at all those previous thoughts. While convinced that you were terminal, you took care of yourself and followed a wellness program. So fear helps to change, to reach out, and to take care of yourself. The problem with fear is that you may have been told by your parents when you were growing up to not be afraid. Some individuals were downright forbidden to be afraid. That can make someone crazy. It is called self alienation. One becomes cut off from his or her feelings and basic instincts. One cannot even rely on his- or herself when needed the most—when an individual is sick.

Fearlessness is simply the ability to be with your fear and not reject it. Your fear is a good friend, and when it is acknowledged, honored, and examined in detail, this is an act of courage and health.

> *To be in good health means not only to be successful in coping with reality, but also to enjoy the success; it means to be able to feel alive in pleasure and in pain; it means to cherish, but also to risk survival.* (Illich, 1976, p. 128)

The role of the therapist is to contact, guide, and help clients renegotiate their pain. You make a mistake when you think you should or can eliminate it, especially if it is chronic. Often pain is seen as the enemy—it must be eradicated. You have developed all kinds of aggressive therapies that neither enrich the patients nor heal them. The context used is manual therapy. There are many techniques, myofascial, cranial, Rolfing, that can create physical change. The usual pattern is for a therapist to take many workshops in different modalities. So the patients receive a little of this and a little of that, which may further promote their confusion. These techniques can overstimulate the autonomic nervous system and cause emotional discharge to occur that is unintegrated. These responses must be properly guided, so the nervous system can complete the pattern and reorganize. Reorganization is the ability of a system to produce new physical patterns as a result of internal regulation in response to change. In order for this to occur, the physical release of energy must be utilized in the viscera as well as the soft tissue system and not dissipated. So a release must go out as well as in to the body. It is through the soft tissue, the viscera, and the central nervous system that one reorganizes and renegotiates pain.

The viscera hold the deeper feeling level of the organism. "I have this gut feeling," "give me your gut feeling," "speak from your heart" are qualities one craves from others and often finds challenging to do yourself. The problem with emotions is that one rarely fully experiences them completely and accurately. Parents were not always the best role models. Often boys are encouraged to deny their fear and sadness and the girls to suppress their anger and individuality. "Little girls shouldn't make noise when they laugh," or shouldn't get angry, and so on, are statements that many parents make to their kids. So individuals grow up emotionally delayed and confused about how to express gut feelings. This is why you want to utilize the energy of soft tissue release, move it into the viscera—to wake up your gut brain. It takes time, patience, and loving kindness. Your own therapeutic process has been ongoing for many years now, and you may feel like you are just starting to scratch the surface of your deep emotions to really look at them. Do so with a fear of the unknown. Spend time in therapy working on your inner rage. Maybe the depression of a degenerating disc in your neck left you unable to do bodywork, your life's career. That was very painful, rewarding, and at times, very humorous.

Pain is the enemy of culture. The ability to experience it has been expropriated by pharmaceutical medicine and the notion that someone other than yourself has the answer and the power to heal it. "Medical civilization tends to turn pain into a technical matter and thereby deprives suffering of its inherent personal meaning" (Illich, 1976, p. 189). Your illness is wasted unless you are transformed by it.

You should not merely objectify pain. It is rich with subjective experience, meaning, and learning. Why is it good to take away someone's pain? This should really turn your head around, especially in your approach to orthopedic patients. It is something you need to consider as manual therapists. It raises the question, "How can I help this person?"

CHAPTER 17

Psychological Issues in Manual Therapy

All manual therapy has the potential to evoke psychological issues. Although research is conducted, regard to the physiology of soft tissue dysfunction and its release, the psychological issues that are ever present in the interaction between therapist and client, are largely overlooked, ignored, or forgotten. When these issues are acknowledged, they can just as easily be mishandled. This article is a brief description of the issues that are most often present between the patient and therapist in a manual therapy practice. The core of these issues are traditionally called transference and countertransference. They are a naturally occurring phenomena between client and therapist. It is a two-way street. Freud felt that the therapist represented an authority or power figure to the patient like a mother or father, and the patient would therefore transfer feelings about his or her parents onto the therapist. The therapist willingly takes on this power. This also applies to the therapist. The patient represents the same figure in reverse—a daughter or son, and so forth. Therapy may involve coming to a resolution of deeper self or family conflicts through this transferring and countertransferring of hidden, unresolved, or unconscious problems. More recently, the meaning of these terms have been expanded to include any projection of a disowned part of the self that occurs in the therapeutic relationship. So, during one session, one may see a male therapist as an angry father, then an innocent son, then an alcoholic boss, or perhaps even a fantasy figure from literature like a warrior or a saint whose story or myth one grew up with or dreamed about.

The practice of manual therapy brings clients who are struggling with their bodies. They enter the office with many hopes and expectations of you and the therapy you provide. When these expectations are unrealistic and unfulfilled, the transference and countertransference intensifies, which gives rise to psychological issues such as resentment, anger, ignorance (why me?), acting out (hysteria, compulsive behavior like drinking), or blurring the boundaries by wanting to socialize with the therapist, forgetting to pay, no-shows, tardiness, and so on. Usually, manual therapists have had little training in communication skills, boundaries, ego defense mechanisms, transference, and psychological ethics. Third parties are often present that could lead to more confusion such as the front desk: secretaries, telephone operators, business office clerks, invisible insurance adjusters, and referring physicians. This buffer zone of paraprofessionals and others becomes an extension of the therapeutic relationship and often contributes to the confusion that prohibits health and healing. Probably you cannot remember how many times patients have come in for a session and spent the first 10 minutes of the session complaining about this person and that person in the chain of office personnel that they had contact with between the last session and now.

One of the best antidotes to negative transference is deep listening. You need not react to the complaint, but simply acknowledge the patient verbally and move on with your work. Sometimes you may repeat what clients say to you. Place yourself in the client's position and say something like, "Gee, if that ever happened to me I'd be pretty upset too." This is not patronizing the client, but rather empathizing with them. Empathy simply means to feel your way into the client's reality, to extend your senses (sight, hearing, smelling, etc.) toward the client.

Business practices often spill over into psychological issues. Appointment keeping, payment for treatment, and no-shows often highlight frustration and confusion between the client and the therapist. The first contact between the therapist and client can be the most important. Boundaries are set, physically and emotionally. The more clarity you can bring to this first interaction, the more you can eliminate tardiness, no-shows, complaining about in-house procedures, and so on. This allows the focus of the interaction to occur in your treatment room. It is not uncommon for therapists to have clients sign agreements acknowledging all the office and business procedures of the clinic. Massage therapists find these issues to be more challenging than physical therapists. The majority of legitimate massage practitioners in this country have little or no business training, and may enter the profession for self-growth and are burned out from a previous career. Massage therapists are aligning themselves more with standard clinical practices, which will lock them into the same frustration and cycle of iatrogenesis that permeates the physical therapy world. Iatrogenesis is defined as physician-induced illness. In other words, the massage therapist becomes part of the problem, exacerbates it, and falls back on medical referrals and third-party payments to keep the cycle active. This is negative countertransference. Healing relationships rarely occur out of this scenario. To treat pain, eliminate symptoms, and attempt to cure the patient does not significantly assist the patient in his or her healing process. A Jungian psychologist once told me that only bacon gets cured.

You are sometimes inwardly confused with how much you talk to clients about your personal life. The issue is called self disclosure. The rule of thumb to use is to always speak from your experience, and not someone else's unless you acknowledge the source. In other words, you may have a neck/disc problem similar to the client's, and you can share your history, and so on, but then recommend a solution or an exercise that you have never tried, and make it sound like you have. It helps to say, "I've not tried this exercise before, but I heard it is really good for your condition." There is a common lie in manual therapy that since the research supports such and such a regimen for recovery, that therefore, everyone that fits that diagnostic criteria will benefit from the regimen. It rarely happens. This is the bane of managed care, that patients can fit into a recipe from a cookbook.

Sex is one of the biggest issues facing a manual therapy practice. Contact is skin to skin and is often confused with sexual intimacy. The largest ethical issue traditionally facing therapists is having sexual contact with clients. This can cover a whole range of behavior that includes improper touching, dating clients, having lunch, and sleeping with clients. When sexuality is confused with intimacy, it will shape the session time with the client. Active fantasies will define the way you touch the person, how often you recommend treatment, and even affect your primary relationship at home. Touching clients meets a fundamental human developmental need. This is well-documented. As a child, you need to be stroked, hugged, caressed, and touched in a loving manner. It is a need that, if unfilled, will stunt or diminish your psychological growth for giving and receiving affection. The need for affection is often confused with sexual intercourse. That is why a manual therapy practice is always meeting a psychological need as well. Already within the first minutes of your treatment, you have listened to clients unconditionally and touched them nonthreateningly. This can be an experience that happens infrequently in your life and can easily be confused with your sex drive and passion for a loving relationship.

When a client removes any or all of his or her clothing, it causes a natural embarrassment, a sense of vulnerability. This is intimate and not sexual. Embarrassment and vulnerability are big issues for many patients. These are called boundaries. They are often transgressed in your life. How many times did you hear your parents say, "grow up, big men don't cry," or "you shouldn't be feeling that. Big men don't *feel* that way," or a mother telling her daughter that "little girls shouldn't get angry," and so on. Children's feelings and emotions are constantly undermined by these statements. Feelings of embarrassment and vulnerability are powerful and need to be honored. If the therapist can honor his or her own feelings, then he or she can honor the clients'. There is a trust that inner feelings will be valued and not discounted. This sense of intimacy in the relationship allows for healing to occur. Now you have not only listened to the client and touched him or her, but also *allowed* him or her to feel what he or she is feeling, without judgment or invasion of boundaries. You have not discounted his or her feelings like so many instances before. Intimacy is associated with having your feelings and then expressing them in a nonjudgmental environment. Body work and manual therapy generate many feelings for the patient. Slowly and gradually over a period of time, a client becomes comfortable with your touch, his or her body, and the feelings connected with his or her body. A teacher once said, "healing is a process, not an event." Healing arises out of the client/therapist relationship and not any particular technique you employ on the client. This is true in the field of psychotherapy, and it is true for manual therapy.

The main styles or expression of negative countertransference (your projections and interpretations onto clients) are arrogance, aggression, and professional distance. Manual therapeutics that do not respect the nervous system's ability to integrate and reorder itself from trauma will drive the trauma deeper, both psychologically and physiologically.

The neurosis of the dedicated health professional consists of maintaining proper clinical distance. The field of massage therapy as well as physical therapy has a strong clinical objective bias. People do not heal with objective, scientific, verifiable data or when they lay behind a curtain for 20 minutes with hot pads and an ultra sound. This is palliative. Yet many clinics in this country are organized that way. This is not discounting the need to stabilize an orthopedic injury or post surgical trauma at all. Rather, these styles of working and approaches to physical therapy often fail to recognize dignity in the body/mind connection and fail to reflect a sane environment. An environment of peace and tranquility is a major contributing factor to the health and well-being of all human beings. The peace and tranquility of a therapist and his or her office is a major antidote to negative countertransference. The first thing to recommend is to provide therapists and their clients with access to a locked, private, quiet treatment room, free from any interruptions, where a patient could be treated for a minimum of an hour. Try it just once a day. Every therapist gets to treat for one hour a day without interruption in a quiet environment. Ultimately, the therapist has a much greater responsibility to manage his or her countertransference, knowing the importance of healthy advertising, a realistic environment, and a sane connection with his or her own self.

The most consistent question asked is, "How should I respond to a client's emotional responses from body work?" Often the questioner is afraid of the responses he or she has seen. It is also indicative of the nature of the therapies being taught now to therapists around the country. Such modalities as myofascial release, cranial work, Rolfing, and visceral manipulation are very potent and evocative therapies. Autonomic discharge, psychophysical unwinding, and emotional catharsis are commonplace. This leaves a big gap in the practitioners' experience because they are not accustomed to seeing it or facilitating it. Then there is a commonly held false assumption by bodyworkers that they can take a weekend workshop in facilitating somatic emotional release and that will solve the problem. It is simplistic and mechanistic. This is just more negative countertransference. Manual therapists are faced with two challenges here. The first one is the basic sense of inadequacy that everyone feels when the client does not improve. This sense of insecurity leads therapists to take more workshops on how to fix the client's physical problem without looking at him- or herself. The second challenge is that many therapists do not know how to handle their own painful emotions or to even recognize them when they come up. This can be very problematic for a therapist. You have more to learn and gain from the clients than they do from you. You model a way of being with your emotions for clients. When you know who you are and where the painful edges of your emotional immaturity are located, then the client senses that. When it comes to emotional release work, an old Southern expression from Alabama is recommended, "Seek not, forbid not." If you choose to work with clients' emotions, you need at least 150 hours of psychology, an M.A., M.S.W., or Ph.D.

Therapists who work with others' bodies would be well advised to take trainings in self-help and self-growth. There are self-help support groups and counseling readily available for anyone wishing to understand his or her confusion and conflicting emotions. It is a well-known principle in open systems theory that if one member of the family gets better, everyone else will change also. So if you want clients to get better, do something to better yourself. Working with emotions involves a cycle of first: recognizing the emotion; second: experiencing it (not acting it out);third: expressing it; and fourth: working to problem solve. This is the cognitive dimension of emotional release work that is forgotten by the somatic-based therapies. Is it realistic to think that a client will experience a permanent change in his or her well-being from being unwound or rebirthed without professional follow-up, especially if the emotional event is linked to developmental, psychomotor, or cognitive deficiencies?

Finally, take responsibility for your emotions and your own actions rather than feeling victimized by yourselves and others. When you are the victim, you go through cycles of dissonance by thinking you did something wrong. You withdraw, you feel sad, then you feel anger. But anger is linked to a cognitive component of feeling wrong. That starts the whole cycle over again. The process of healing involves a wholehearted ownership of yourself and your life. This is the greatest gift you could mirror for clients and ultimately teach them. You teach them by acknowledging their feelings and emotions and giving them permission to feel what they are feeling. This can be done very simply. When you see tears in a client's eyes, you can ask, "Do you want me to continue my work or should we take a break for a while?, "It is okay to feel what you are feeling," and so on. Placing your hand over his or her diaphragm or on his or her abdomen, over his or her chest or under his or her neck very lightly can be a signal for the client that it is okay to explore his or her feelings and begin to allow them. Just say, "You're doing fine—stay with it," or "That's good, see if you can allow yourself to feel here" (wherever you happen to be placing your hand).

Clients and you are part of an open system. Illness occurs in the whole context of a person's life, not just the body. This means that all factors, that is, lifestyle, diet, psychology, anatomy, spirituality, and so on, play an equally important role in the ability to experience health and healing. It is important to recognize these issues as they come up and to manage them effectively. Active listening (mirroring), boundary setting, owning one's emotions and feelings, and providing a peaceful office are the beginnings of creating an environment for the mutual exploration of health and healing.

CHAPTER 18

Types of Body Shock by Michael J. Shea, Ph.D.

This talks about different categories of shock and also when your ability to work with trauma becomes thwarted. Shock is a restriction of motor patterns and a restriction of the sensory field. It is a result of a breach in the barrier against overstimulation. Over time these breaches activate defense mechanisms. What does that mean? Shock causes dissociation (Putnam, 1993). There is an alternation or suspension of thoughts, feelings, or behavior so that for a period of time, your consciousness is suspended and other information is not associated or integrated. When the organism receives a shock, there is a thwarting response. First there is a physical obstruction of arousal activity. Usually one tries to suppress anger even when one is justified, so an individual clenches his jaws, tightens his flexors, and so on (Feldenkrais, 1949). Second, there may be a simultaneous arousal of two or more responses. When you perceive fear or shock, it activates the fight-or-flight response. You have a tendency to want to fight, but you may also want to run. Guess what happens? You freeze. That is an inhibitory response. The physical obstruction of the arousal activity is that inhibitory response. The other typical response is death-feigning or sham death (Ludwig, 1983). You go slack in your tissue and take on a posture of resignation. One response leads to hypertoned tissue, and the other to hypotoned tissue. There are also combinations that occur (Levine, 1992).

These two responses are a choice the organism makes, and one usually prefers one or the other throughout life. If the type of shock allows for fight or flight, then the pattern may complete itself. However, if you do not fight or flee, your central nervous system goes on overload and begins to select a response for you. That leads to a thwarting response of arousal activity. Well, guess where that goes? It goes into your myofascia. You freeze. "I'm scared stiff." The flexor system of the body stiffens. When the flexor system of the body does that, your blood capillaries are being squeezed. That leads to ischemic compression in the soft tissue. It causes a decrease in oxygenated blood, and the cardiovascular system backs up. It can lead to high blood pressure or angina. You go to your doctor, and you get medicine for it, yet you continue to stay in a dysfunctional family, or you continue to stay in an abusive relationship, or you choose to stay in a high-stress job with a boss who is an ogre. You continue to lead a lifestyle that is high strung, that leads you to the need for surgery, or into a sequence of accidents, that is, cervical whiplash, so now you really are physically dysfunctional. That is how one handles shock. The body is the dumping ground for many problems.

Sham death responses lead to passivity in the tissue and the personality. Sham death is a dissociative state that results from trauma or shock that is irreconcilable or overwhelming (Ludwig, 1983). Dissociation experiences that persist may lead to post traumatic stress disorder (PTSD) or even multiple personality disorder.

The surgery itself, or the cervical whiplash itself, is what you are dealing with when you get your hands on clients. You are not trained or equipped to work with the psychological implications. When you get your hands on, and you begin doing manual therapy, you see all sorts of whistles and bells go off in the autonomic nervous system that are indicating that you are on track in terms of activating or arousing the ability to respond appropriately (potentially) to that shock. You help organize a new response, you help renegotiate the old trauma, and you help integrate to a higher level of functioning after the activation and sympathetic discharge begins. This creates a space for self-regulation.

Here is a little about the different causes of shock. When I got out of college, I was commissioned as an officer in the army, and the Vietnam War was just winding down, so I was stationed in Frankfurt, West Germany. This was supposedly peacetime. I worked in a large office building at a major European command headquarters. I lived across the street in a ground-floor apartment for bachelor officers. I went over to the officers' club one day, and parked my car next to a very large terrorist bomb. I got out of my car and went into the officers' club and turned a corner into the dining room and the bomb went off. I was covered in rubble (along with everybody else). The man who was just parking his car in back of my car, a lieutenant colonel, was killed. My car was completely destroyed. This was a massive high-intensity shock with blood horror. I saw the lieutenant colonel with his head decapitated and partially in the back seat of my car. I have spent many years in psychotherapy as well as receiving a lot of bodywork to recover from the sensory overload of that shock. I have included an essay as an appendix to this chapter that thoroughly describes my inner journey from the experience and ultimately having chronic post-traumatic stress.

These types of experiences create an environment for dissociation and dissociative phenomena that is post-traumatic stress disorder. Post-traumatic stress disorder is another legacy of the Vietnam War. There are some grim statistics about the soldiers that actually survived the Vietnam War in terms of suicide, crime, and mental illness. One needs to be more pragmatic. It is unknown how many physical therapists or massage therapists are seeing Vietnam veterans, but therapists are seeing post-traumatic stress syndrome all the time in orthopedic injuries, surgeries, and so on. The American Medical Association in 1995 named virtual violence as a major source of stress and anxiety. Virtual violence is the violence on TV, in newspapers, or the movies. One can now experience post-traumatic stress disorder from watching TV. An individual keeps his nervous system in a state of arousal with no completion. Think about it. Even 5 years after a cervical whiplash, some patients develop post-cervical whiplash syndrome, which is a first cousin to post-traumatic stress. Getting in a high-speed automobile accident, or even a low-speed at 15 to 20 miles an hour, is very violent. Your nervous system undergoes a shock. That is what happens in a massive high-intensity situation like that, whether it is a bomb, a car wreck, or constant television. It takes years to undo that. The combination of cranial work and soft tissue work is a big part of providing relief from that shock.

There are many varieties of shock trauma, including such high-intensity events as neurological insults at birth or closed-head injuries. There are degrees of how the body's shunting mechanism inhibits the damage. As an adult, one is much more easily able to handle a big shock than a small infant can because of shunting mechanisms. An adult can take the energy from a shock and put it into the viscera, the central nervous system, the skeleton, the joint spaces, or into the heart. The human organism is extremely sophisticated. The trauma will show up in the soft tissue. It will show up as high tone or low tone or chronic pain or chronic fatigue or myofascitis or fibromyalgia, and so on. And because every macrophage is connected to a sympathetic nerve, ultimately the immune system will suffer (Arnason, 1993).

The second type of shock is surgery. Surgery is a very large shock to the organism whether it is a tonsillectomy or a C-section. There exist some interesting experiences working with women who have had C-sections. They have gotten myofascial release as well as psychotherapy. They found that the nervous system was thwarted in not being able to have a vaginal delivery. In working with some severe traumatic discharge patterns, since the body was not able to complete a normal delivery, years later during myofascial release, the reflex action of the vaginal delivery in the tissue starts to complete itself. You might want to think about it when you are doing pelvic work for unrelated circumstances with a woman who has had a C-section or working on the scar tissue. It is important to clear this scar tissue. Adhesions can adversely affect the hip flexors, the viscera, and pelvis floor.

The third type of shock is inescapable attack. The amount of physical, sexual, and emotional child abuse in this culture is astounding. Keep your eyes open when you are working with clients. There are numerous signs that the body gives off as a result of that abuse. Often the abuse is forgotten and is secondary because it is so far away in the past or masked by other physical or developmental problems. Their reporting symptoms are primary. The secondary process is very important. It is the client's psychological process. The medical model misses this. You do not have to be trained as a psychologist to see secondary process happening in the patient. What this is trying to teach is to observe autonomic functioning. This is preverbal and precedes the symptoms that you are presented with from clients. This secondary process in the autonomic nervous system is actually more important. The most important cue is to be mindful, especially when working on the adductors. Please do not work the adductors until you have had several sessions with the client. When you do work on the adductors, and you need to at some point because they are deep fascial anchoring of the spine, do so carefully and respectfully. Go slowly and ask for feedback. Keep looking at the client's eyes.

There is an interesting distinction here when escape, which is inhibited either physically or internally, is perceived as a lack of resources. This is when you get attacked, and you feel you do not have the inner strength or the wits to deal with it.

A four-year-old kid was all alone one day and walking down the street. A Doberman attacked him and bit his ankle. He never told his parents. He never told anybody about it. That stayed with him for 20 years. He was absolutely terrified of dogs when he was a kid growing up. He always heard about those rabies shots and the long needles in the belly. Yuck! All that pain! So, he never bothered to tell his parents He was bitten by a dog, but every time a dog barked at him for the next 20 years, he would have an anxiety attack.

May be you have noticed that you have been in a lot of shocking situations. Everyone has. You cannot underestimate the body, and all it has been through and the thread of relationship between life's events and your symptoms.

Number four is physical injury. You see a lot of physical orthopedic injuries. This includes diseases and hospitalizations where people have been immobilized, as well as some types of auto accidents. You can be a passenger and get sideswiped or you can be the driver and do a few spins on an icy road. It is just staggering how the central nervous system and your body respond to that stress. You change your breathing. You change your blood chemistry. You change your immune system. You change your entire neurophysiology. Hardly any component of the body is left unscathed by chronic stress. In this context, stress causes significant changes in soft tissue tone, as well as postural tone. Bodywork helps the central and autonomic systems decompress from trauma quite effectively. Exercise is also very important. Nutrition is very important. Prayer and meditation are also very important (Dossey, 1993; Kabat-Zinn, 1985).

There is a fifth category, which is failure of physical defenses. These are falls. When you trip and fall off of a curb or steps, it is differentiated from physical injury because it involves more vestibular functioning. Much of the central nervous system is oriented toward upright posture; when you brace yourself for a fall, it is easy to break a bone or bruise a joint, and so on. Many orthopedic injuries are the result of falls. This is where myofascial release is particularly beneficial because of the tightening and shortening that occurs in the fascia.

Finally, you have environmental, cultural, and psychological shock. Here is an example of culture shock. When I got out of the army, there was a recession in the early 1970s, and I did not have a job. I had been a high school English teacher. I had a good job in the military. However, I ended up working as a merchant seaman because I was just tired of being in unemployment lines for almost a year. That was really hard for me. That in itself was a shock. I shipped out as a merchant seaman, and I got placed onboard a ship where alcoholism was rampant. Only half the crew could read or write. For the first time in my life, I saw people sign their paychecks with an "X." That is how they got paid. I went through estrangement, repulsion, and withdrawal for six months. I was completely shocked. I did not know how to be in that system. I did not know how to interact or be social. That is culture shock.

There are very common psychological shocks. If you look at the statistics of some of the most stressful events in people's lives, you will find marriage and divorce right at the top. Marriage is stressful. Divorce is very stressful. There are many types of psychological shocks. You can live with someone who has a process addiction to his or her emotions; people who all of a sudden are irrational. You do not know when it is coming out.

There is also environmental shock. There is always a certain intensity when you shift environments from the familiar to the unfamiliar. It is not what your central nervous system is accustomed to processing. This causes tension in the body, in soft tissue, and/or viscera.

This mentions several other types of organic shock.

> *Shock is a vascular change resulting from assault or injury to the body. Any condition that reduces the heart's ability to pump effectively or decreases venous return can cause shock. Hypovolemic shock (hemorrhagic) results from fluid volume loss after severe hemorrhage or loss of plasma in burn patients. Treatment includes administration of plasma or whole blood. Neurogenic shock is due to generalized vasodilation, resulting from decreased vasomotor tone. The reduced blood pressure causes poor venous return to the heart and hence poor cardiac output. The decreased vasomotor tone may be due to spinal anesthesia, spinal cord injury, or certain drugs. Anaphylactic shock*

> *accompanies a severe antigen—antibody reaction such as occurs in an incompatible blood transfusion. Cardiogenic shock is the result of extensive myocardial infarction. It is often fatal, but drugs to combat it are sometimes effective.*
> (Mulvihill, 1980, p. 136)

It is not unusual at all for clients to experience mild or moderate anaphylactic shock from prescription medications and food allergies. It would be valuable to screen clients for food allergies and to make sure of all known side effects from any medications they might be taking. Even mild anaphylactic shock will effect tissue tone. Some medications may also cause neurogenic shock. Because these symptoms may be masked by the reporting symptomology or orthopedic problem of the client, a careful review of their intake form of medication and dietary history would be valuable. Food allergies are much more common with the denatured type of food in the west. Seventy percent of the world's population is lactose intolerant, and yet in the United States, milk and dairy products are consumed by the majority of the population. This was all made clear along with the resulting problems with dairy and excess sugar by the Select Senate Committee Reports on Human Nutrition and Dietary Goals for the United States. This document may still be available from the U.S. Government printing office in Washington, D.C. It was originally published in the mid-1970s.

The autonomic nervous system is like a radar system. The perception of shock or the perception of fear is initiated and perceived by the autonomic nervous system. The central autonomic network (CAN) is a network of nerve pathways that regulate the autonomic nervous system in the brain. In many ways, the hypothalamus coregulates the autonomic system. But there is a switchboard in the nucleus tractus solitarius located in the brain stem that channels sympathetic input to the limbic system and especially the hypothalamus. Therefore, the nucleus tractus solitarius and hypothalamus are said to coregulate the autonomic nervous system (Low, 1993).

When you orient yourself to fight or flight, inhibition or shunting, one of the first things you do is contract your diaphragm. You also change the tone in your flexors and extensors and go through very complex physiologic changes systemically. This is well-documented in the work of Hans Selye, so I will not spend more time with these specific dynamics (Selye, 1976). Here is a brief list of some of the dynamics of the general adaptation syndrome that Selye describes:

- increased heart rate
- constricting of blood vessels of viscera and skin
- sweat production increases
- respiratory passageways are widened; rate of breathing increases
- contraction of spleen
- decrease in enzyme production by digestive organs
- adrenal medulla increases secretion of epinephrine and norepinephrine
- blood sugar level increases as the liver converts stored glycogen into glucose
- kidney activity is cut back because of decreased blood flow to the kidneys
- retention of sodium/shunting of potassium, which is excreted with urine
- increased glucocorticoids accelerate protein catabolism
- thyroid stimulation results in the catabolism of carbohydrates

- liver stimulation results in the catabolism of fats
- increased glucocorticoids slow wound healing because of diminished connective tissue formation
- loss of potassium ions results in dehydration of the cellular cytoplasm

Generally you handle most shocks in your life. Some of them get the best of you. The internal perception of some shocks produces altered states called dissociative phenomenon (Putnam, 1993). These states are: amnesia, depersonalization, derealization, identity disturbances, absorption, or enthrallment experiences. Dissociation also includes spacing out, inattention, and some transient sensations. Depersonalization is an out of body experience or near death experience. Demonic, spirit, and trance possession states are widespread as dissociative phenomena. Depression, anxiety, and hyperarousal are states of dissociation. These symptoms must be addressed in body therapy, as they are regulated via the limbic and hypothalamic areas of the brain. They have a strong influence on the soft tissue of the body, and any of these dissociative symptoms will accompany shock trauma.

Out of these states of dissociation, you create change. You renegotiate the experience and self organize. In many cultures the ones who have had great shocks and healed themselves are chosen to be the healers to help guide others. This is called the wounded healer paradigm (Campbell, 1949). Often shock becomes an opening for realizations or spiritual crises (Grof & Grof, 1990). There is a potency to responses that is yours alone. You suffer a death and live to tell about it. Illness is wasted unless you are transformed by it. Many healers have had near death experiences or serious illnesses.

Everything is crystal clear for just a brief moment to people who undergo a shock. That is what is called the healing image. It is the color of the bark on the tree you just hit. It is the rain splattering the windshield upside down on the highway. It is the feel of warm blood trickling down your face. It is the slow flickering of the overhead fan you are staring at as you are being sexually abused. That is the healing image and a reference point for clients. The appearance of a healing image during a session means to slow down the pace of your work, particularly if you can switch into any soft-style indirect work that has impact on his or her nervous system, like cranial work. You have to realize the nervous system is oriented around inhibiting sensory data. The spinal cord is swimming in endogenous opiates. As a therapist, you are on a fishing expedition to find the healing image where the organism perceived a death and build back out from there. Sometimes this is a verbal process for clients. Very often they do it on their own internally with their own images and metaphors, and you help utilize the charge autonomically from the soft tissue (sympathetic) back into the viscera (parasympathetic) deep inside.

There was a woman who was overdosed with anesthesia when she was in the hospital for pelvic inflammatory disease. She was pregnant, and it distended her so much that they had to perform an abortion. Then they overdosed her, and she nearly died. She spent three days in a class. She was going through more pelvic discharge at night and then the disorientation from the memory of the drugs during the class. She was very strong and brave. The therapist just kept encouraging her like a coach, and at the end of the three days, she was exhausted but integrated. Her body and emotions became synchronized from talking to the group and integrating cognitively. The process started on the first day of a cranial class from looking up into the ceiling lights that were just like the surgical amphitheater. That healing image opened her up to renegotiating that trauma.

It is unclear how long it takes somebody to get over any particular shock. Healing is a process, not an event. Everybody has their own time cycle by which they will heal. Any physical trauma is going to be tied into the physiology and psychology of the person's life at that very point. Your input may shift the illness to a less debilitating level.

Manual therapy allows you to locate people's physiological boundaries. This is very good information for you as well as for them. You can reeducate people once you have found their boundaries (Katherine, 1991). Much autonomic phenomena goes unacknowledged because the perception internally is one of either, "I am out of control," or "This looks stupid," or "I feel silly." These are the thought-forms that go on with autonomic discharge, as well as "I am embarrassed," "What the hell is that?" "Now I am sweating," "Oh, I feel clammy," "That feels weird." You, the therapist, are participating in that process. It does not make any difference what technique you are using. The autonomic system gets activated and may discharge while you are doing bodywork. It is your responsibility to be informed and prepared to assist in an appropriate manner.

Any time you lay your hands on a client, you are catalyzing autonomic responses. It is doubly important that when you apply direct technique, like myofascial release, that you know what it looks like if the nervous system cannot integrate, organize, or negotiate the level of energy and input you are using. Do not as an instructor say, "Use five pounds in technique number two." What you could say is, "Use pressure slowly, incrementally." Then watch if the client holds his or her breath, the eyes glaze over, he or she cries or disassociates. Then you are into the autonomic nervous system, and you are accessing more information about that person and that trauma than was previously known, by you or them. The next step is to slow down or stop at that point and observe what the nervous system is doing with that information. Slowing the input or stopping it completely will most likely affect a slower restimulation of traumatic sensations and perceptions. This slower response can allow the client's shunting systems to reorganize trauma that originally occurred rapidly—so rapidly that a major component of the traumatic memory may consist of general sensory overload. Next you are going to help the client integrate trauma through his or her breathing and the space or container of safety that you are creating in your office. This is called soft seeing.

The bottom line is very simple: stop working and let them breathe for two to three cycles of respiration. Take a break for a minute and just say, "I see your feet are breaking out in a sweat. Can you feel that? How do you feel?" They are just really simple questions. "Where do you feel yourself in your body right now?" If somebody says, "I feel numb" or "I do not feel anything" I say, "Pick a part of your body that you feel right now. Any part will do." And I make a game out of it. The autonomic stuff is often unconscious. It is hypothalamic and visceral. Keep your eyes open to their breathing, their eyes, and their thoracic outlet. These areas have most of the autonomic nerves. You are an observer and a guide. Use your language carefully to bring about cognitive integration. Rather than asking "What do you think about that?" try "Where do you feel that in your body?" Stay body-centered with the client.

Peter Levine (1991) works with a five-stage model when treating shock trauma. The first stage is sensation. Your touch is deliberately slow because you are bringing sensation to the client and the area that needs healing. Sensation leads to imaging. As mentioned earlier, this goes back to what Levine calls the healing image. The healing image is the central or focal point of the original shock trauma that the client orients his or her body around. The way a client orients his or her body with injury and illness involves unconscious behavior. This is the realm of secondary psychological connections that fuel the primary responses in the body. They are inseparable. Primary and secondary do not mean levels of importance, but rather that which is known—the body, and that which is unknown in your behavior. These three—sensation, image, and behavior lead to affect. Affect refers to feelings, perceptions, and emotions. Affect is a physical or neurological event associated with shock trauma. Affect is always there, and sometimes affect moves into catharsis, which is reliving the shock trauma with a strong memory. It is not necessary to relive or remember shock trauma to heal it.

Meaning-making is the last stage of the Levine model for somatic experiencing. Meaning-making is the intrinsic capacity of the human psyche to make sense of life on a moment-to-moment basis and the shock trauma that catapults one into the realm of the unknown and mysterious. You make meaning by the metaphors you live by (Lakoff & Johnson, 1980; Olds, 1992). You make meaning with the stories and myths you grew up with (Jung, von Franz, Henderson, Jacobi, & Jaffe, 1964). You are participating in clients' meaning-making with manual therapy. If you open your eyes and slow down, you may help clients bring new meaning to their problems that is hopefully more intelligent.

Indications of Shock

- Abrupt changes in affects and behavioral states, for example, sudden, flattening of affect, emotional outburst, abrupt changes in behavioral activity
- Sudden exaggerated startle lasting for a long duration—may be somewhat masked by voluntary inhibition or performance unwinding
- Body sensations of numbness, immobility, and restlessness
- Stuporous gaze or fixed gaze without recognition—particularly when startled or aroused
- Exophthalmus "big eyed"
- Amnesia for events or loss of affect in describing probable charged events—dissociation
- Rigid immobility or waxy flexibility in muscles

- Parkinsonian-like tremor

- Particular hyper- or hypotonic muscles not appropriate to general developmental pattern of body map

- Abrupt loss of vocal behavior

- Fainting—dizziness

- Autonomic indications: Fixed pupils (very large or very small); dryness of eyes (mydriasis); simultaneous sympathetic or parasympathetic (masking) such as decreased heart rate with peripheral vasoconstriction, that is, cold hands; appears relaxed but with high heart rate

- Suspicion (conspiracy theories), panic-anxiety, agoraphobia, agitated depression, most psychosis, and multiple personalities

- Breath holding—hyperventilation

Most of the prior examples are made more instable with stress—particularly multiple target vectors, muscular, skeletal, visceral, central nervous system, and endocrine.

Causes of Shock

- Massive high intensity trauma

- Inescapable attack

- Physical injury

- Failure of physical defense

- Environmental, cultural, and psychological

Thwarting—Situations

- Absence of indispensable stimuli following intense arousal
- Physical obstruction of aroused activity
- Simultaneous arousal of two or more incompatible tendencies

Primary Responses to Thwarting (Somatic)

- Perseverance—persistent approach and adjustment
- Impulsivity—capricious choice of response
- Threshold intention movements—initial element of response
- Ambivalent posturing—elements of several responses
- Tonic immobility

Primary Responses to Thwarting (Autonomic)

- Alimentary—salivation increase or decrease, urination, defecation
- Circulatory—pallor, flushing, genital vasodilation, fainting
- Respiratory—changes in breathing rate and amplitude, gasping, sighing, panting
- Thermo-regulatory—sweating, pilomotor activity
- Lacrimatory—weeping

Secondary Responses to Thwarting

- Irrelevant behavior
- Immature responses
- Loss of responsiveness
- Intense approach and adjustment

This chart was made from notes at a Peter Levine, Ph.D., workshop and his two books (Levine, 1997, 2010).

CHAPTER 19

Working with Shock Physiology

Bodyworkers are really good at observation skills. You stand people up and give a very detailed explanation of where the hips are and where the shoulders are and where the bony and soft tissue relationships are and where the lack of symmetry is. What is often missing is observing the nonmechanical components of structure (Keleman, 1989). The way in which you look at the nonmechanical components of structure is by looking at arousal states in the autonomic nervous system, and in particular how the sympathetic and parasympathetic nervous systems discharge in rhythm with each other. You look at how this autonomic nervous system goes into flux and how it has balanced itself between sympathetic dominance and parasympathetic depression. You look at how the body can handle this charge or arousal. Remember that the sympathetic nervous system regulates two systems: all of the soft tissue in the body and every blood capillary as a sympathetic innervation. The sympathetic nervous system also talks bidirectionally to the immune system via macrophages, T-cells, some B-cells, lymph tissue, and the thymus gland. Parasympathetic depression is the visceral response. This is referring to the viscera, to the enteric system, to the vagus nerve in the cranium, and to the sacrococcygeal plexus in the sacrum.

The other term to think about is that instead of observing the autonomic nervous system, you are tracking it. You could facilitate the process by which the autonomic nervous system contributes to self-healing and self-regulation of the organism. What this means is to pace your work in terms of the level of input to the client. Pacing means slowing down and taking a break every few minutes. You cannot keep up constant input to the organism because you will overload the autonomic nervous system. Most clients are already overloaded in their autonomic system. You could drive the trauma deeper—first into the cardiovascular system and then into the digestive system. You may irritate the pathology. Pacing and tracking have to do with slowing down, stopping, and looking. In terms of technique, it means allowing for two or three cycles of respiration in between each application of a technique. You could say that respiration is the glue between the physical and emotional responsiveness of the organism. In this way you may avoid retraumatizing the client and dissociating them.

Trauma does not come out of the body. You do not get rid of trauma. Rather, trauma gets integrated. There are three words that are important—trauma gets integrated, trauma gets organized, and trauma gets renegotiated within the central nervous system. It gets organized or integrated or renegotiated to a higher or lower level of functioning depending on a number of factors. They are lifestyle, family system, environment (environment meaning social system, educational system), and physical constitution. You can give a child all the help he or she wants, but if he or she has to go back to a dysfunctional home and his or her parents are alcoholics, it is going to be really hard to renegotiate a trauma to a higher level of functioning without healthy support.

The last factor is involved with a reeducation. This is a strong attempt to reeducate the organism and the central nervous system to go to that higher level, both functionally and structurally. You work on the structure to give it congruence to support function. Improved function will disintegrate without a congruent structure that includes a flexible autonomic nervous system. This may also include, but is not limited to, psychotherapy, movement reeducation, proper nutrition, a new job, a new spouse, and so on. A new spouse or job may happen, but one does not work toward that. You work to support improved relationship skills. Therapists have many opinions about what the client needs to do in their personal life, some of which is perfectly valid. However, these reactions are countertransference issues, especially in a manual therapy practice (Wolfstein, 1998). You can make specific recommendations or even give homework for the clients; however, you can lead a horse to water but you cannot make him or her drink atone of the biggest problems in the body therapy community is an obsessive drive to overload the client with things to do between sessions. Try to decrease the load on the client. When giving homework, attempt to distill it down to one thing. What is the one thing, one small thing that a client might try between sessions? If you make a recommendation that will take more than 5 or 10 minutes a day, its execution is based on careful consideration of a client's ability to manage his or her time well and his or her level of commitment. Most clients come back and either do not do their homework or have failed at it and feel guilty. Find the one thing, the one small thing, that may make a difference over time. This concept is called trimtabbing. A trim tab is a small rudder placed on the large rudder of oceangoing ships. It was found that by turning the small rudder first, it would influence the direction of the ship more quickly than by turning the large rudder first.

You have the capacity to organize sensory input (a neurological insult that a cerebral palsy child might have, or an orthopedic trauma, a surgical trauma, or cervical whiplash, etc.) and motor output to a higher level of functioning. This is the meaning of integration (Ayers, 1979).

You have a shunting mechanism in your autonomics. The level of input you give to the system reaches a given capacity, and then shunting moves into other systems of the body. When you lay your hands on people, you are accessing their myofascial system. There is a hierarchy within which the myofascial system, or any system of the body, can handle energy. Each system takes so much input and then places it somewhere else in the body. The hierarchy goes something like this: you go from the myofascial system to the cardiovascular system to the alimentary system. You have gone from the two major systems of sympathetic dominance—from the myofascial system into the cardiovascular system. That is where stress goes—stress response. Then you go into the visceral digestive system. You know how many people have visceral digestive problems, as well as backaches and cardiovascular disease? Then you shunt into the hypothalamus and get into endocrine problems because of elevated cortisol, and so on. There is also a chronic disturbance of thermoregulatory and homeostatic mechanisms, like chronic sweating, chills, and shakes. For a thorough discussion of autonomic disorders, see Low (1993).

The mediating factor between these systems are the fluid dynamics in and around each cell. The fluid systems of the body get stressed. What you are attempting to delineate is how the body handles shock, how the body receives and works with a shock, and how it comes to resolution. Shock is a restriction of the sensory field and the deletion or restriction of motor patterns. Shock causes dissociation, which prevents integration from occurring.

Here is a list of the indications for shock. These are also dissociative phenomena.

1. Abrupt changes in affect and behavioral states are the substrate of emotion and feeling. All at once there is a flattening of affect. You will be in the middle of a session, and the tone will drop dramatically, or it will reverse. You will be working with someone, and then all of a sudden you will get this big spike in activity. They will be real talkative, or they will start getting real fidgety. They could start crying—whatever it might be. But, there will be an abrupt switch over, an abrupt change in behavior, either very quiet or very active.

2. A sudden exaggerated startle. The client will start shaking uncontrollably, or they will start self-splinting. Clients might start hyperventilating or get into chronic tetany. That is an indication of shock. You have either shocked the body or you have accessed an old shock in the client's body. This is good news. This is what you are looking for. You evoke it and then help guide it. Be careful of nongenuine unwinding. This can be called performance unwinding because what you see when people begin to unwind is a very dramatic neuromuscular or gross motor unwinding, which can be completely avoiding the core-level issue. In their shock, they keep going around and around the issue. You see that in athatoid children. They keep leaking energy out their appendicular skeleton without being able to access their trunk—their middle. They are fixated in their sympathetic response, unable to access their parasympathetics.

3. Body sensations of numbness, immobility, and restlessness. If you have a client describing to you, "I feel numb. I cannot move. I cannot move that limb," or if they get real fidgety every time you work on them, that is a chronic dissociative pattern that they get into. Once again it means you may be accessing an important shock and trauma.

4. Clients get a blank gaze in their eyes or stare at something without recognition, especially when they are startled or aroused. You see that a lot in survivors of sexual abuse. In work of resolving psychophysical trauma in adults, there is a strong pattern of disassociation. When a child is physically, sexually, or emotionally abused, it is such a shock to the system that he or she cannot integrate it. They disassociate. You see him or her staring off into the distance. You could be deep into his or her psoas,

but he or she has disassociated and does not feel a thing. Learn to recognize that look in the client's eyes. Check in verbally to confirm conscious presence. There may be a long pause before you get a reply or you may have to check in verbally several times before they reply.

5. Exophthalmia; a bug-eyed look where the eyes are wide open, like they have just seen the ghost of Christmas past. Clients often come in looking like this.

6. Amnesia for events or loss of affect. This is classic in child abuse as it manifests in adults. Children do not remember, but the adult may suddenly remember. It is not at all unusual to be in the middle of working with someone, and they remember the event. They remember being raped by an uncle. They remember the car wreck at the age of three where they got bounced around in the back seat. This is a very special, almost sacred space you have created where the client feels safe enough to open up. Memory is always mixed with imagination (Hillman, 1990). The memory is an event that is taking place right now in his or her body. The trauma is in the way you remember the event right now.

7. Hypertoned immobility in the tissue. If you have a client whose tone keeps rising while you are working, you are headed in the wrong direction. You have also accessed that shock/trauma, which is valuable. It means you are on the right path, and you have to choose a different strategy or style of work. Instead of working with the problem areas, work to support the areas in a client's body that are strong.

8. Clients begin to fasciculate. That is a low-level shaking or trembling in the muscles. This is a sympathetic

response. Vagotonic parasympathetic responses are different. They are sudden jerks in the spine, headaches, and nausea. Smiling also activates the parasympathetic system. When a client is having a sympathetic discharge that is not accompanied by strong emotional content, ask the client to smile to see if that fits the release that they are having. Very often a discharge is just a release of energy and excitation that actually feels good. By smiling, the client has the opportunity to raise vagal parasympathetic tone which is very beneficial (Gellhorn, 1960).

9. Fainting and dizziness. This is self-explanatory.

10. There are different types of psychological indications: depression and chronic depression, as well as panic and anxiety. If your mother has anxiety attacks, you may develop anxiety attacks. May be you always thought that you were the only one in the world that got them, then you realized how you learned them. You inherit behavior from your parents. This is beginning to be well-documented in psychology (Bradshaw, 1988).

You do not have to look at whether this shoulder is higher or not. You can look at the eyes, you can look at the face, you can look at the breathing response, and you can listen to his or her voice. Those are the main keys that you need to know in terms of accessing the client's secondary process. A lot of times structural problems are the primary process from a medical point of view. The client walks in complaining of shoulder pain or low back dysfunction, whatever it might be, and that is primary. Then as you give the body some input, all of a sudden he or she is staring off into the distance or describing a numbness in his or her body. This is secondary or the background material coming to the foreground. It is your entree into the shock trauma system. It is the cause, and it is the therapeutic leverage that will relieve the symptomology most comprehensively when used in conjunction with appropriate interventions. So you see, secondary process is actually very important, but you have to work through the primary reporting symptoms first to integrate the secondary process.

The direction that you take is to help get the client into a quiet place and to help access his or her core. Core means his or her digestive-visceral, vagal system. It is right in front of his or her spine. That is the place where people can go inside and resolve trauma. You help return the client to parasympathetic dominance (Criswell, 1989). The idea here is that you are guiding the organism. You are carefully observing an event, and then you are helping to guide it and direct the energy inward so that clients quit leaking that parasympathetic energy out to the appendicular skeleton. Clients can then go deeper into their central nervous system and/or their viscera to resolve trauma if they have the time and space, the love and support of mindful therapists. This love and support becomes a container or boundary system for the client to do his or her healing (Keleman, 1986).

The bottom line is that the nervous system perceives a shock as a death-like experience. "Oh, my god, I am about to die!" Unwinding and emotional discharge can be part of the process. To resolve it you guide that person to go inside and figure it out for themselves. Unwinding and emotional discharge are intermediate steps. You can lead a horse to water, but you cannot make it drink. The client must participate in his or her own health. This can be learned, and it is part of your responsibility as a health professional to help educate clients. They also need motivation, which requires a safe, trustworthy environment in which to live and work (Maslow, 1970). You must remember that client/therapist relations are full of ethical considerations (Purtilo, 1993; Taylor, 1995). Somatic-emotional unwinding clients is one of the most ethically charged situations in the profession today.

That means setting up circumstances, so that clients can access and discharge tone—and then let them organize and resolve it inside. When a client goes deep inside to integrate, it is called a state change or a phase transition. You see that all the time in your work. You will be working, and all of a sudden there is a state change. The tone is dropped, something is going on, and you can sense it. The room gets quiet, the client gets quiet. Even you get quiet. Something happens. *Bingo!* That is it. They have dropped out of their sympathetic arousal reaction. The client has gone into their hard-disk drive. They are reprogramming. You have taken the old software out, and they have a chance to plug in new software. To get congruence in a new pattern usually requires repeat treatments.

That is the beauty of state changes. It is like an ocean tide. Allowing someone to go into a state change where they are real quiet, then come out and go through a period of reeducation at the end. This has a rhythm to it (Rossi, 1986; Weiner, 1992). Sometimes that involves movement work or referring the client to a psychotherapist. A lot of bodywork is psychologically provocative. That is ethically challenging. Over 60 percent of Americans are overweight and out of touch with their bodies. The statistics are staggering. There are 80 million alcoholics in this country, and each one seriously affects the lives of seven other people. Three out of five women (two out of five men) have been sexually abused. Then, that person has cervical whiplash and maybe even gallbladder surgery. The dysfunction gets cemented in the body like that. It is a multiple shock psychologically and physically (Lowen, 1958).

Finally, how to resolve shock must be addressed. First you must discuss the notion of looking for motility and not mobility. Motility is the rhythmic response of tissue to the intrinsic rhythms of the body like heart, breath, cranial, and so on. When you feel the cranial rhythm, you are feeling the motility of the cranial rhythm. When you are feeling a rib cage, you are also feeling the motility of breathing. It is a qualitatively different level of palpation. You use the soft tissue to listen to the inside of the body. Motility is the rhythmic response within the myofascial system to intrinsic pulses of the body (pulses meaning respiratory, cranial, vasomotor, vagotonic—there are a wide variety of pulses in the body). They all have a palpatory feeling within the tissue. You have been trained for years and years to release a joint space and to feel when a muscle or a fascial plane releases. Try to begin to shift—not only your observation skills, but also your palpation skills. Most people do not know when a true release comes because they are still oriented in a very linear fashion around a joint space opening up or a muscle softening. This is fundamentally different. You can feel motility with myofascial release by slowing down and tuning into intrinsic tissue motion. There is motility within the motility. There is an intelligence that is expressed by the motility of the fascia.

Other ways exist to help a client through depression and anxiety. These are so common now in culture and for so many reasons. Maybe you will refer someone to an occupational therapist so they can learn to balance their checkbook or manage their time better. Some clients need to learn very simple relationship and parenting skills. Classes to learn these skills are available much more so today than ever before. Another example is clinical Ericsonian hypnotherapy. Clinical hypnotherapy is an excellent way to work with anxiety and phobias as well as many other problems. Also prayer and meditation or pastoral counseling are perfectly wonderful, especially for devout Christian clients. You live in a day and age where the causes and conditions of people's physical problems are quite complex. While the research in touch therapy is growing by leaps and bounds, do not forget that you have a mind that is intimately connected to your body. At some point the mind may need treatment.

CHAPTER 20

Myofascial Release: Blending the Somatic and Orthopedic Models by Michael J. Shea, Ph.D. and Dale Keyworth, P.T.

> Although used for many decades, little has been documented or written about myofascial release (fascial release) concepts. The system is a complex form of soft tissue manipulation based on the operator's ability to monitor functional, anatomic, and neurologic influences. Developed by American osteopathic practitioners, MFR [myofascial release] led, with important exceptions, to clinically pertinent, fascially-based discussions almost exclusively in the osteopathic literature, but only after 1950. (Ward, 1993, p. 225)

Myofascial release is usually taught at the basic level as a positioning technique or stroke intent applied to soft tissues of the body. These approaches may be classified as direct techniques such as Rolfing developed by Dr. Ida Rolf or indirect techniques such as muscle energy and strain counter-strain (Greenman, 1989). As in cranial osteopathy and its derivatives, the skill of the practitioner will often determine if the technique is direct or indirect. Positioning techniques include strain and counter-strain and muscle energy techniques. When joint biomechanical rules, called arthrokinematics, are integrated into the treatment, the treatment is a myofascial manipulation. Regardless of the direct or indirect myofascial techniques chosen, the basic question remains: How should these different techniques be organized?

The techniques are usually formed by the development of a strategy at the beginning of each session. This strategy is based on feedback from the client and clinical observations about the client's physical and emotional demeanor. A key to forming the strategy is developing appropriate and insightful skills of observation. What is observed about the outside world, and especially about another's body, is formed by 80 percent neuroassociation and only 20 percent from the retina of your own eyes (Varela et al. 1992). The implications of this are clinically significant. It is quite possible to have many thoughts triggered by looking at a client. Therapists may have preconceived notions about the way a body should look, move, and perform that do not relate to the individual client. These preconceptions will influence the quality of the clinical work both consciously and unconsciously.

A fundamental requirement of structural myofascial integration is acknowledging that observational skills at times feel incomplete and confusing. Observational skills need to be based on the discipline of self observation, with careful attention to the practitioner's own sensations, feelings, and inner thoughts in relationship with what is being observed. It has been stated by Heisenberg in his uncertainty principle that you cannot observe something without changing it. Just by looking at a client in a clinical mode changes the client. Therapists have many nonclinical thoughts about the client (This person is attractive, this person looks sad, etc.) and themselves (I'm tired, I'd like to go home, etc.). These nonclinical thoughts and personal sensations are usually considered an epiphenomenon (Sheets-Johnstone, 1992). Sensations and feelings are subjective and often discarded as something that has little relevance to the client-therapist relationship in a treatment session. However, all personal thoughts and feelings are important and impact upon the relationship therapists have with their clients.

The primary mode of learning how to see a client is through the symmetry or lack of symmetry in a client's musculoskeletal system. The therapist looks at a client and notices that one shoulder is higher, one leg is shorter, one hip is higher, or the head is not on the center line. From an embryological and developmental point of view, there is no such thing as symmetry in the body (Blechschmidt & Gasser, 1978). Individuals all have intrinsic, organic, right-left, front-back, top-bottom splits in symmetry (Dychtwald, 1977). The body develops in a spiral pattern that mimics the double helix pattern of DNA and RNA (Dart, 1950). Observing symmetry gives information about orthopedic trauma, but looking more closely below the surface develops what is called soft seeing. Soft seeing looks for how the central, autonomic, and enteric nervous systems have integrated or mediated shock trauma into the soft tissues. Soft seeing observes skin color, postural tone, rapid eye movements, patterns of muscular contraction, movements (fasciculations) such as shaking and trembling, changes in breathing, voice patterns, and sweating. These signals indicate that the client is having a sympathetic nervous system discharge and may be integrating some aspect of their trauma into their healing process. Clinically, these increased sympathetic arousal signs will rebound into the parasympathetic nervous system. The parasympathetic nervous system becomes more dominant as the client utilizes new found flexibility in their autonomic nervous system. Soft seeing starts the moment a client walks in for the appointment and becomes critical as you start to use myofascial release.

Recognition of the improvement in postural tone caused by the parasympathetic nervous system response to treatment is a clinically effective result. This recognition is a reassurance to the clinician in his or her treatment. The signals mentioned above can easily be seen regardless of whether the client is sitting, standing, or lying on the treatment table. These autonomic discharge patterns and the affect left over from shock trauma can be integrated by acknowledging them verbally and kinesthetically. These small spontaneous movement patterns should be encouraged from the extremities toward the midline or if they start at the midline, then encourage movement toward the extremities. When these fasciculation occur, the therapist slows their input and lightens their touch. This allows integration to occur and avoids retraumatizing the client (Levine, 1997).

The goal is to encourage treatment organization that allows clinicians to see patients and clients with new eyes and new hands. The clinician can view each client with a sense of wonder and appreciation, that sees past the client's exterior asymmetries and appreciates the unspoken message of inner emotional and physical being. Heightened emotional and physical awareness of the clinician's own personal subjective experience is vital to treatment. Recognizing that both the clinician and patient may be embarrassed at the client's being seen in his or her underwear, for example, does impact the treatment, especially in a multicultural practice. This embarrassment or confusion may be an opportunity for the clinician to view his or her own feelings so they can move into a blending of clinician/patient energies to achieve an organized and integrated healing process. Healing processes are a collaborative effort and are a function of relationship as much as any technique that is employed.

There are three elements of the clinician's personal subjectivity: the first is embarrassment, which means acknowledging thoughts and feelings such as disgust, boredom, curiosity, desire, fear, and compassion. The second element is the wonder and uniqueness of the physical and emotional qualities of the client. Finally, the third element relates to the aesthetics of balance rather than symmetry. Myofascial release is an art form, and the therapist is a sculpture. These form the basis for organizing a treatment plan for the client. This is the beginning of a somatic understanding of myofascial release.

> *Somatic process work looks at how a client has structured his past experience and how he can destructure it to form a new structure. When a client's way of reaching out and coming back to himself is*

> *thwarted, his form gets repressed or distorted. Then he projects his needs onto the world in stylized ways. A central focus of somatic process work is disorganizing these muscular-emotional patterns. This is called grounding, a somatic, psychological, and emotional process which involves imagination, thought, feeling and action. . . . The essential goal of somatic process work is for a person to experience his life in its bodily and emotional shape with the feelings that are present and how they are organized, and then to know the associated meanings and memories. To know your own forming process is to know how you have embodied experience.*
> (Keleman, 1986, pp. 63, 80)

When practicing myofascial release, it is important to understand various biological principles and characteristics of the fascial system. The first principle is that fascia acts like an organic crystal with an electrical, chemical, and magnetic communication system (Oschman, 1993). An orthopedic injury or shock trauma to the body changes this bioelectromagnetic configuration at the cellular level, because compression of a crystalline substance, fascia, produces a change in the electrical field. This change produced by compression of a crystalline substance is called the piezo-electric effect. Fascia is a semiconductor, thus manual therapy can change or enhance this bioelectromagnetic configuration dramatically.

There is a continuous fascial sheath surrounding every muscle, organ, and bone of the body. The superficial fascia is one continuous layer of fascia that is subdermal. The retinaculum of the feet and ankle contain thick fascial bands that form a bridge between the deep and superficial fascias of the body. The connective fibers in this fascia include collagen, elastin, and reticulum (Oschman, 1984, p. 7). There are four categories of collagen fibers. Type I is found in loose, dense connective tissue that is the most commonly treated type of fascia. Type II collagen is found in hyaline cartilage. Type III collagen is found in the fetal dermis and lining of the arteries. Type IV collagen is found in the basement membrane of cells (Grodin &

Cantu, 1992). A continuum of structure and communication travels from every cell nucleus in the body via the microtubules of each cell basement membrane wall to the collagen fibers of the fascia itself (Grodin & Cantu, 1992).

The other important component of all connective tissue is the ground substance. Ground substance is a viscous, amorphous gel with a high water content. Ground substance contains collagen fibers and various cells like fibroblasts. Histologically the fibroblasts are the primary secretory cells in connective tissue, existing in the collagen, elastin, reticular, and ground substance. It is a function of the ground substance to diffuse nutrients and waste products. The ground substance also acts as a mechanical barrier to invading bacteria and other microorganisms. Together the various collagen fibers and ground substance are called the extracellular matrix (Grodin & Cantu, 1992).

The primary components of ground substance are glycosaminoglycans substance and water. Glycosaminoglycans were referred to as acid mucopolysaccharides in the older literature. Glycosaminoglycans can be divided into sulfated and nonsulfated groups. The nonsulfated group, which is predominantly hyaluronic acid, binds water. Connective tissue is approximately 70 percent water. A change in water content of the connective tissue affects the critical interfiber distance in the ground substance. When there is an injury to the soft tissue, the ground substance appears dehydrated, and the collagen fibers bind together forming a gel-sol relationship. In an orthopedic trauma or related stress to the fascial system, the dehydration of the ground substance causes the interfiber distance between the collagen fibers to shorten. In addition, this dehydration becomes a glue or gel. At this point, the collagen fibers begin to crosslink and form a much tighter bond to protect the body. Manual therapy and purposeful movement have the potential to rehydrate the ground substance, which turns it back into a solution and subsequently returns the collagen to a healthy interfiber distance. This is what is meant by the gel-sol relationship. Clinically the skin feels tight and dry. All of these changes in the ground substance are mediated by the bioelectromagnetic configuration of the fascia.

The second principle is: fascia acts like a fluid system in response to stress and strain. Stress and strains on living biological material is described by biorheology in terms of shear forces and tension. Fascia exhibits non-Newtonian type fluid/semi-solid, chaotic behavior because of the tensile properties of collagen. Stress to the fascial system may be unpredictable in its effects. Injury to the fascial system causes systemic compensations throughout the body, not just locally. It is difficult to predict where compensatory patterns will occur. Somato-visceral and viscero-somatic interactions are not in register segmentally in the spinal cord. Visceral influences converge on the cord along with somatic influences and may span as many as five segments of the spinal cord. This leaves many possibilities and multiple sites for injury to be distributed through the body, not just in the fascial system. Chronic knee pain may adversely affect the bladder, liver problems can affect the eyes, and so on. Nociception and the processing of pain has a pervasive influence in the body and central nervous system and may cause what is generally referred to as an adaptive response. Thus a minor injury to a system that is already in an adaptive response may cause a reaction quite larger than normal (Willard & Patterson, 1992). A client may have a sub-clinical bowel problem, sprain their ankle and become constipated, develop headaches, and lose sleep.

The third biological principle is: the body is capable of building more fascia than it can remove. Scientists feel that the need for rapid, adaptive patterning is part of the evolutionary process. Any injury to the soft tissues must undergo the process of shortening and tightening to heal. These changes in collagen binding begin to occur within 20 minutes of an injury or sustained postural distortion. The longer the distorted, immobile position is maintained, the more collagen fibers will crosslink to form newer, tighter bonds. These bonds will spread within days to adjacent joints above and below the site of the injury. The fascial binding affects the entire body since the fascia has multilayered continuity from top to bottom and outside to in. This may account for some of the reflex activity seen in myofascial pain syndromes (Travell & Simons, 1992). Recognition of how the body has compensated or adapted to trauma and injuries around the midline or core of the body is an important treatment principle in myofascial manipulation.

Strategies for integrating the fascial restrictions are based on the functional divisions of the fascial system and how contact is made with this system appropriately. The easiest way to enter the system is at the level of the superficial fascia. Only after freedom is achieved in the superficial layers and enlivened with broad light contact can the deep fascia be engaged (Rolf, 1989). The deep fascia is considered to be the layer continuous with and surrounding the deep postural support muscles. These muscles include the tibialis and peroneal group in the lower leg, the interosseous membrane between the tibia and the fibula, the adductor complex, the ilio-psoas-diaphragm group, the mediastinum, the pectoralis minor and subscapularis, the scalenes, the pterygoid muscles, and the meninges.

At a practical level for time management during a myofascial treatment, the superficial fascia is engaged for the first 20 to 30 minutes followed by the deep fascia for 10 to 15 minutes. This is followed by more superficial fascia reorganization before concluding by organizing the integrative fascia. The integrative fascia is all the paraspinal fascia. Organizing the paraspinal fascia has a direct positive biomechanical effect on the brain and spinal cord as well as the vascular and lymphatic vessels of the spine. It carries the work done throughout the body directly into the spinal cord.

With multiple treatment sessions, a trilogy of planning and organization is possible. Several options are available when doing a series of three treatments. One trilogy might begin with a session on the lower extremities and pelvic girdle, followed by a second session on the shoulder girdle and upper extremities, with a third session specific to the axial midline and spine. Other trilogy options might focus on three sets of three sessions: three superficial fascia sessions, followed by three deep fascia release sessions, and conclude with three paraspinal integrative sessions. The combinations possible with this planning model are numerous.

There are three additional practical organizational concepts. The first is that the dorsal and ventral fascias of the trunk migrate laterally under stress or from injury. This means that the fascia over the abdomen and rib cage is to be moved up and back toward the spinal column to restore postural tone. Then the fascia over the spinal erectors is moved medially and down from trapezius to sacrum.

The second concept is that the best access to the superficial fascia of the client's body is along the coronal plane when the client is side lying. This coronal plane in side lying is like a tailor's seam in a good suit and is the point where all fascial "seams" converge. The bony margins, such as the iliac crest, are an ideal place to separate the many fascial planes as they converge. Key structures are the lateral malleolus, head of the fibula, greater trochanter, crest of the ilium, ribs, head of the humerus, the mastoid process, and parietal (bone) ridge.

Third, separate the fascial septa between the muscles that are not gliding over each other properly. The fascial septa are the bags or containers of the individual muscles. Injury causes the septa to bind to each other, thus restricting motion. Next, free the various retinacula on the legs, arms, trunk, and spine. The posterior serratus muscles act as retinacula for the erectors. The retinaculum has the greatest potential for binding because the superficial and deep fascia merge there. Releasing these deep and superficial fascial junctions is essential for free movement of the fascia.

An important treatment concept for integration is called periodic disengagement. As the clinician applies significant direct pressure to the client's body, it is crucial for the practitioner to take their hands off the client's body and observe the client's respiration for two or three cycles. This disengagement allows the client to integrate the soft tissue work into their nervous system and permits the clinician to evaluate the cumulative effect of their treatment. Without periodic disengagement, the risk of retraumatizing the client occurs as the autonomic nervous system fails to integrate the tissue work (Levine, 1997). Give the nervous system time to integrate the soft tissue release. The autonomic nervous system is not always in register with the soft tissue because of adaptive responses because of stress and injury (Patterson & Howell, 1989).

Periodic disengagement is the ideal time to scan the client from head to toe. Close attention should be paid to the eyes, skin color, postural tone, facial expression, set of the jaw, tension patterns in the scalenes and capital flexion, position of the trunk (elevated or depressed), shaking or trembling in the extremities, contraction in the rectus abdominus, and stillness in the pelvis. These are all signs of how the sympathetic nervous system is integrating or failing to integrate your input. Usually these indicators are telling you to slow down, take a longer break between pressure applications, and lighten your pressure. Request that the client give you feedback about the quality of your touch by asking if they are comfortable. Then pay attention to how they respond with any affect rather than the words they use. Ask a client where they are sensing the work and not how they are feeling the work. Feeling is a loaded word and is preceded by body sensation. Reassociate the client to body sensation. In addition, use the word *allow* frequently, that is, "Can you allow this to go into your back?," "Can you allow this to go into your hip?," and so on.

Chronically immobile, frozen tissue is indicative of shock and/or trauma (Levine, 1997). Tissue that has a waxy flexibility, that seemingly is in a state of resignation with little tone is also an indication of shock trauma. It is important to check with the client verbally from time to time concerning comfort level and body sensation. During shock trauma, the organism has two basic choices when flight or fight is thwarted. The first choice is called inhibitory freezing. The body becomes rigid and stiff with terror. Soft tissue shortens and decreases circulation (Levine, 1992). When left untreated, this condition armors the body and causes psychological changes to occur (Reich, 1945).

The second choice around shock/trauma is death feigning. This response is hardwired into the nervous system and is seen quite often in the animal world. It is also known as playing possum. The body collapses into a defenseless posture, and the soft tissue becomes soft and spongy. This condition also has psychological correlates and usually is seen in endogenous depression (Herman, 1997). Together these two conditions are habituated into the myofascial system and will respond best to slow, patient, skillful touch, and communication. These myofascial palpation skills are based on quality, quantity, depth, direction, and duration. Slow, purposeful movement participation by the client is critical in restoring the function of depressed tissues. Clinical failures result from a lack of engaging the client consciously. A morphic focus seems relatively ineffective compared with a tonic focus for depressed tissue.

The hallmark of direct myofascial work is a flow that moves from contact with the breath and active movement followed by increased awareness, interaction, and finally integration. Contact with the client begins preverbally and intuitively as they make the appointment, and thoughts and feelings are generated in the therapist. Contact then moves to a stage of touching the tissue itself. Next, the therapist observes the client's breathing as well as his or her own breath. Ask the client to breathe slowly and deeply into the point of contact. Rapid breathing indicates the client is not accessing his or her intrinsic muscles and may be in hyperarousal with the autonomic nervous system. Therapists need to check in with their own breath and be aware of any changes in their own respiratory pattern. The therapist's breath is an important feedback system, not only about personal internal states, but also those of the client through a type of therapeutic transference. Next ask the client to move the joint closest to where you are working. As Ida Rolf once said, "Take the tissue into its anatomically correct position and ask for movement." This movement facilitates integration into the nervous system and facilitates release of tight tissue. It also helps soften the occasional intense sensation.

Throughout these stages, there is a growing awareness of the pattern of tension in the client. As the awareness of the client is enhanced, the possibility for psychological integration is also present. Awareness is a function of an increase in sensation in the motor sensory cortex in the brain as well as perceptions and feelings networking throughout the brain and body. Awareness ultimately evolves into a consciousness of an organized meaningful whole experience. This is called gestalt formation (Perls, 1951). It is essential to cultivate awareness by attending to your own feelings and sensations. By modeling this to the client, a much deeper level of integration and functionality is facilitated. This may simply mean that the client walks better at the end of the treatment or that they have just released a month's worth of anger. There is no way of predicting how the client will work with their own awareness. This is where skill with myofascial release intervention comes into play. Intervention is being made in a complex pattern that the client has formed in their soft tissue system. This pattern has a significant relationship to other systems of the body, as well as the sociocultural context within which the client currently lives and historically how they sustained their shock trauma. Intervention in the fascial system has the potential to impact many levels of a person's life both quickly and dramatically. Understanding basic principles and following subjective somatic insights rather than merely applying a technique offers greater opportunity for successful clinical outcomes.

This is a somatic model of myofascial release. The evolution of experienced meaning for the client is impacted not only by who you are and the environment, but also, at a very pragmatic level, by your pacing, depth, and direction of touch. These qualities of the somatic model help reduce transference and countertransference issues between the client and the therapist. The client is empowered when the therapist models a new way of touch and is sensitive to the environment. Direct technique cannot be applied without significant personal awareness and subtle observation skills. The client needs to be verbally empowered to tell you when to stop, when to slow down, and when to back off. Therefore, it is important to carefully educate the client about attending to their subjective sensations rather than ignoring or suppressing them. In this somatic model, emotional process may occur but is a secondary gain in the relationship between the client and therapist (Jackson, 1994). The best therapeutic motto is "Seek not, forbid not." It is not within the scope of practice of any touch therapist to deliberately provoke emotional responses in the client. However, bodywork and especially myofascial release seem to have emotional release as a byproduct of the intervention. When the client experiences a genuine emotional release, the therapist maintains an empathetic posture and allows this response to be integrative by paying attention and allowing the response. What is of primary importance in the somatic model is therapeutic insight, emotional clarity, and sensitivity (Johnson, 1986).

What is also important is proper contact. Contact is more than just talking and touching the client. "To be in contact, we need to be grounded, have adequate boundaries, enjoy unrestricted breathing, have access to feeling, and have the intention to be present. To be fully present, reflects a functional and durable sense of self" (Conger, 1994, p. 56). Making unbiased, unconditional, nonjudgmental space for the client's reactions is essential. These treatment principles are the foundation for how to see and touch the client. Myofascial release is the medium. The main tools are the therapist's own responses, the coldness or warmth evoked by the client, and the understanding of such responses in dealing with the client

(Keleman, 1986). The end result clinically is a more rapid healing response in injured tissue.

This article originally appeared in *The Clinical Bulletin of Myofascial Therapy*, Vol. 2, No.1, published by the Haworth Medical Press.

RESOURCES

Holly Pinto, LMT, BCTMB
Owner and director of the Body Therapy Center
and School of Massage, Ltd.
Four Executive Woods Court
Swansea, IL 62226
618–239–6400
www.thebtcsm.com
therapybtcsm@aol.com

Michael J. Shea, PhD
13878 Oleander Ave.
Juno Beach, FL 33408–1626
561–493–8080
www.michaelsheateaching.com
info@michaelsheateaching.com

Tim Shafer, MS
Biodynamic Craniosacral Therapy Instructor, Certified
Advanced Rolfer
3500 JFK Parkway, Suite 209
Ft. Collins, CO 80525
970–229–1925
www.indianpeaks.biz
rolfer@indianpeaks.biz

Valerie A. Caruso, LMT, BCST, NSCA-CPT
Excellent Bodywork, Inc.
Biodynamic Craniosacral Therapy Instructor; Continuing Education in Pre- and Perinatal Massage, Infant Massage, and Myofascial Therapies
North Palm Beach, FL 33408
561–283–3404
www.excellent-bodywork.com
Valerie@excellent-bodywork.com

REFERENCES

Arnason, B. G. W. (1993). The Sympathetic Nervous System and the Immune Response. In P. A. Low (Ed.), *Clinical Autonomic Disorders* (pp. 143–154). Boston, MA: Little, Brown and Company.

Ayers, J. A. (1979). *Sensory Integration and the Child.* Los Angeles, CA: Western Psychological Services.

Bechara, A., & Naqvi, N. (2004). Listening to Your Heart: Interoceptive Awareness as a Gateway to Feeling. *Nature Neuroscience, 7*(2), 102–103.

Blechschmidt, E., & Gasser, R. (1978). *Biokinetics and Biodynamics of Human Differentiation: Principles and Applications.* Springfield, IL: Charles C. Thomas.

Blechschmidt, E., & Gasser, R. (2012). *Biokinetics and Biodynamics of Human Differentiation: Principles and Applications, Revised Edition.* Berkeley, CA: North Atlantic Books.

Boissonnault, W. G., & Bass, C. (1990). Pathological Origins of Trunk and Neck Pain: Part 1—Pelvic and Abdominal Visceral Disorders. *Journal of Orthopaedic and Sports Physical Therapy, 12*(5), 192–202.

Booth, R. J., & Ashbridge, K. R. (1993). A Fresh Look at the Relationships between the Psyche and Immune System: Teleological Coherence and Harmony of Purpose. *Advances, 9*(2), 4–23.

Bradshaw, J. (1988). *Bradshaw: On the Family.* Deerfield Beach, FL: Health Communications.

Camilleri, M. (1993). Autonomic Regulation of Gastrointestinal Motility. In P. A. Low (Ed.), *Clinical Autonomic Disorders* (pp. 125–132). Boston, MA: Little, Brown and Company.

Campbell, J. (1949). *The Hero with a Thousand Faces.* Princeton, NJ: Princeton University Press.

Cassidy, C. M. (1994). Unraveling the Ball of String: Reality, Paradigms and the Study of Alternative Medicine. *Advances, 10* (1), 5–31.

Conger, J. (1994). *The Body in Recovery: Somatic Psychology and the Self.* Berkeley, CA: Frog.

Conrad, E. (2007). *Life on Land: The Story of Continuum, the World-Renowned Self-Discovery and Movement Method.* Berkeley, CA: North Atlantic Books.

Cottingham, J. T. (1985). *Healing Through Touch.* Boulder, CO: Rolf Institute.

Cottingham, J. T., Porges, S. W., & Lyon, T. (1988). Effects of Soft Tissue Mobilization on Parasympathetic Tone in Two Age Groups. *Journal of the APTA, 68*(3), 352–356.

Cottingham, J. T., Porges, S. W., & Richmond, K. (1988). Shifts in Pelvic Inclination Angle and Parasympathetic Tone Produced by Rolfing Soft Tissue Manipulation. *Journal of the APTA, 68*(9), 1364–1370.

Criswell, E. (1989). *How Yoga Works: An Introduction to Somatic Yoga.* Novato, CA: Free Person Press.

Cunningham, A. (1955). Pies, Levels and Languages: Why the Contribution of Mind to Health and Disease Has Been Underestimated. *Advances, 11*(2), 4–30.

Dart, R. A. (1950). Voluntary Musculature in the Human Body: The Double-Spiral Arrangement. *The British Journal of Physical Medicine, 13*(12), 265–268.

Davidson, R. J., & Begley, S. (2012). *The Emotional Life of Your Brain: How Its Unique Patterns Affect the Way You Think, Feel, and Live—and How You Can Change.* London: Hudson Street Press.

Dossey, L. (1993). *Healing Words: The Power of Prayer and the Practice of Medicine.* San Francisco, CA: Harper Collins.

Dychtwald, K. (1977). *Body Mind.* Los Angeles, CA: Jeremy P. Tarcher.

Feitis, R., & Schultz, W. (1996). *The Endless Web: Fascial Reality.* Berkeley, CA: North Atlantic Books.

Feldenkrais, M. (1949). *Body and Mature Behavior.* Madison, CT: International Universities Press.

Findley, T. W., & Schleip, R. (2007). *Fascia Research, Basic Science and Implications for Conventional and Complementary Health Care.* Munich: Elsevier GmbH.

Foreman, R. D. (1989). The Functional Organization of Visceral and Somatic Input to the Spinothalamic System. In M. M. Patterson & J. N. Howell (Eds.), *The Central Connection: Somato Visceral/Viscero Somatic Interaction* (pp. 178–202). Indianapolis, IN: American Academy of Osteopathy.

Foss, L. (1994). The Biomedical Paradigm, Psychoneuroimmunology, and the Black Four of Hearts. *Advances, 10*(1), 32–50.

Freedman, D. H. (1994). Quantum Consciousness. *Discover, 15*(6), 88–98.

Gardner, H. E. (1983). *Frames of Mind: The Theory of Multiple Intelligences* (2nd ed.). New York, NY: Basic Books.

Gellhorn, E. (1957). *Autonomic Imbalance and the Hypothalamus.* Minneapolis, MN: University of Minnesota Press.

Gellhorn, E. (1960). The Tuning of the Autonomic Nervous System through the Alteration of the Internal Environment (Asphyxia). *Acta Neurologica, 20*(4), 515–540.

Greenman, P. (1989). *Principles of Manual Medicine.* Baltimore, MD: Lippincott Williams & Wilkins.

Grodin, A. J., & Cantu, R. I. (1992). *Myofascial Manual: Theory and Clinical Application.* Gaithersburg, MD: Aspen Publishers.

Grof, S., & Grof, C. (Eds.). (1990). *Spiritual Emergency: When Personal Transformation Becomes a Crisis.* Los Angeles, CA: Jeremy P. Tarcher.

Harman, W. (1995). Exploring the New Biology. *Noetic Sciences Review, Summer*, 29–33.

Herman, J. L. (1997). *Trauma and Recovery: The Aftermath of Violence—From Domestic Abuse to Political Terror.* New York, NY: Harper Collins.

Hillman, J. (1990). *Myths of the Family (Part 1 and 2).* Two audio cassettes. Available from Sound Horizons Audio, 250 West 57th St. #1527, New York, NY 10107.

Hoheisel, U., Taguchi, T., & Mense, S. (2012). Nociception: The Thoracolumbar Fascia as a Sensory Organ. In R. Schleip, T. W. Findley, L. Chaitow, & P. A. Huijing (Eds.), *Fascia: The Tensional Network of the Human Body* (pp. 95–101). London: Churchill Livingstone.

Horgan, J. (1994). Can Science Explain Consciousness? *Scientific American, 217*(1), 88–94.

Illich, I. (1976). *Medical Nemesis: The Expropriation of Health.* New York, NY: Random House.

Jackson, S. W. (1994). Catharsis and Abreaction in the History of Psychological Healing. *Psychiatric Clinics of North America, 17*(3), 471–491.

Johnson, D. H. (1983). *Body: Recovering Our Sensual Wisdom.* Berkeley, CA: North Atlantic Books.

Johnson, D. H. (1986). Principles vs Techniques: Towards the Unity of the Somatics Field. *Somatics, VI*(1), 4–9.

Johnson, D. H. (1994). *Body, Spirit and Democracy.* Berkeley, CA: North Atlantic Books & Somatic Resources.

Jung, C. G., von Franz, M. L., Henderson, J. L., Jacobi, J., & Jaffe, A. (1964). *Man and His Symbols.* New York, NY: Bantam.

Kabat-Zinn, J. (1985). The Clinical Use of Mindfulness Meditation for the Self-Regulation of Chronic Pain. *Journal of Behavioral Medicine, 8*(2), 163–190.

Katherine, A. (1991). *Boundaries: Where You End and I Begin*. New York, NY: Fireside/Parkside.

Keleman, S. (1985). *Emotional Anatomy*. Berkeley, CA: Center Press.

Keleman, S. (1986). *Bonding: A Somatic-Emotional Approach to Transference*. Berkeley, CA: Center Press.

Keleman, S. (1989). *Patterns of Distress: Emotional Insults and Human Form*. Berkeley, CA: Center Press.

Korr, I. M. (1979). *The Collected Papers of Irvin M. Korr*. Newark, OH: American Academy of Osteopathy.

Lakoff, G., & Johnson, M. (1980). *Metaphors We Live By*. Chicago, IL: University of Chicago Press.

Langevin, H. M., & Sherman, K. J. (2007). Pathophysiological Model for Chronic Low Back Pain Integrating Connective Tissue and Nervous System Mechanisms. *Medical Hypotheses, 68*(1), 74–80.

LeDoux, J. E. (1993). Emotional Networks in the Brain. In M. Lewis & J. M. Haviland (Eds.), *Handbook of Emotions* (pp. 109–118). New York, NY: Guilford Press.

Levine, P. (1986). Stress. In M. G. H. Coles, E. Donchin, & S. W. Porges (Eds.), *Psychophysiology: System Processes, and Applications* (pp. 331–353). New York, NY: Guilford Press.

Levine, P. (1991). *The Body as Healer: Transforming Trauma and Anxiety*. Lyons, CO: Ergos Institute (in press).

Levine, P. (1992). The Body as Healer: A Revisioning of Trauma and Anxiety. In M. Sheets-Johnson (Ed.), *Giving the Body Its Due*. Albany, NY: SUNY Press.

Levine, P. (1997). *Waking the Tiger: Healing Trauma*. Berkeley, CA: North Atlantic Books.

Levine, P. (2010). *In an Unspoken Voice: How the Body Releases Trauma and Restores Goodness*.Berkeley, CA: North Atlantic Books.

Low, P. A. (Ed.). (1993). *Clinical Autonomic Disorders*. Boston, MA: Little, Brown and Company.

Lowen, A. (1958). *The Language of the Body*. New York, NY: Macmillan.

Ludwig, A. M. (1983). The Psychobiological Functions of Dissociation. *American Journal of Clinical Hypnosis, 26*(2), 93–99.

Macintosh, J. E., Bogduk, N., & Gracovetsky, S. (1987). The Biomechanics of the Thoracolumbar Fascia. *Clinical Biomechanics, 26*(2), 78–83.

Maitland, G. D. (1986). *Vertebral Manipulation* (5th ed.). Boston, MA: Reed Educational and Professional Publishing.

Maslow, A. H. (1970). *Motivation and Personality* (3rd ed.). New York, NY: Harper Collins.

Maslow, A. H. (1971). *The Farther Reaches of Human Nature.* New York, NY: Penguin.

Morgane, P. J. (1992). Hypothalamic Connections with Brainstem, Limbic and Endocrine Systems. In F. H. Willard & M. Patterson (Eds.), *Nociception and the Neuroendocrine-Immune Connection* (pp. 155–181). Athens, OH: University Classics.

Mulvihill, M. L. (1980). *Human Diseases, A Systemic Approach* (3rd ed.). Norwalk, CT: Appleton & Lange.

Olds, L. E. (1992). *Metaphors of Interrelatedness: Towards a Systems Theory of Psychology*. Albany, NY: Suny Press.

Oschman, J. L. (1984). Structure and Properties of Ground Substances. *American Zoology, 24*(1), 199–215.

Oschman, J. L. (1989a). How Does the Body Maintain Its Shape? Part I: Metabolic Pathways. *Rolf Lines, XVII*(3), 27–29.

Oschman, J. L. (1989b). How Does the Body Maintain Its Shape? Part II: Neural and Biomechanical Pathways. *Rolf Lines, XVII*(4), 30–32.

Oschman, J. L. (1990). How Does the Body Maintain Its Shape? Part III: Conclusions. *Rolf Lines, XVIII*(1), 24–25.

Oschman, J. L. (1993). *The Connective Tissue and Myofascial Systems.* Available from Nature's Own Research Association, P.O. Box 5101, Dover, NH 03820.

Panjabi, M. M. (2006). A Hypothesis of Chronic Back Pain: Ligament Subfailure Injuries Lead to Muscle Control Dysfunction. *European Spine Journal, 15*(5), 668–767.

Paoletti, S. (2006). *The Fasciae: Anatomy, Dysfunction and Treatment.* Seattle, WA: Eastland Press.

Patterson, M. M., & Howell, J. N. (1989). *The Central Connection: Somatovisceral/Viscerosomatic Interaction.* Paper presented at the 1989 International Symposium.

Perls, F. S. (1951). *Gestalt Therapy: Excitement and Growth in the Human Personality.* New York, NY: Dell.

Pert, C. (1995). Candace Pert, Ph.D.: Neuropeptides, Aids, and the Science of Mind-Body Healing. *Alternative Therapies, 1*(3), 71–76.

Pert, C. (1997). *Molecules of Emotion.* New York, NY: Random House.

Pincus, T., & Callahan, L. F. (1995). What Explains the Association between Socioeconomic Status and Health: Primary Medical Access or Mind-Body Variables? *Advances, 11*(1), 4–36.

Pollack, G. (2013). *The Fourth Phase of Water: Beyond Solid, Liquid, and Vapor.* Seattle, WA: Ebner & Sons.

Porges, S., Doussard-Roosevelt, J., & Maiti, A. (1994). Vagal Tone and the Physiological Regulation of Emotion. *Monograph of the Society for Research in Child Development, 59*(2–3), 167–186.

Purtilo, R. (1993). *Ethical Dimensions in the Health Professions* (2nd ed.). Philadelphia, PA: W. B. Saunders Company.

Putnam, F. W. (1993). Dissociative Phenomena. In D. Spielel (Ed.), *Dissociative Disorders* (pp. 1–16). Lutherville, MD: Sedran Press.

Ratner, S. (1979). The Dynamic State of Body Proteins. *Annals of the New York Academy of Sciences, 325*, 189–209.

Reich, W. (1945). *Character Analysis.* New York, NY: Simon & Schuster.

Reich, W. (1997). *Character Analysis* (3rd ed., V. Carfagno, Trans.). New York, NY: Farrar, Straus and Giroux.

Rolf, I. P. (1978). *Ida Rolf Talks About Rolfing and Physical Reality.* Boulder, CO: Rolf Institute.

Rolf, I. P. (1989). *Rolfing.* Rochester, VT: Healing Arts Press.

Rossi, E. (1986). *The Psychology of Mind/Body Healing: New Concepts of Therapeutic Hypnosis.* New York, NY: W. W. Norton.

Rubik, B., Becker, R. O., Flower, R. G., Hazlewood, C. F., Liboff, A. R., & Walleczek, J. (1994). Bioelectromagnetics Applications in Medicine. In *Alternative Medicine: Expanding Medical Horizons, NIH Publication 94-006.* Washington, DC: Government Printing Office.

Ruskin, A. P. (1979). Sphenopalatine (Nasal) Ganglion: Remote Effects Including "Psychosomatic" Symptoms, Rage Reaction, Pain and Spasm. *Archives of Physical Medicine Rehabilitation, 60*(8), 353–358.

Schimke, R. T., & Doyle, D. (1970). Control of Enzyme Levels in Animal Tissues. *Annual Review of Biochemistry, 39*, 929–976.

Schleip, R. (2003). Fascial Plasticity—A New Neurobiological Explanation. Part 1. *Journal of Bodywork and Movement Therapies, 7*(1), 11–19.

Schleip, R., & Jager, H. (2012). Interoception: A New Correlate for Intricate Connections between Fascial Receptors, Emotion and Self Recognition. In R. Schleip, T. W. Findley, L. Chaitow, & P. A. Huijing (Eds.), *Fascia: The Tensional Network of the Human Body* (pp. 89–94). London: Churchill Livingstone.

Schleip, R., Vleeming, A., Lehmann-Horn, F., & Klingler, W. (2007). Letter to the Editor Concerning "A Hypothesis of Chronic Back Pain: Ligament Subfailure Injuries Lead to Muscle Control Dysfunction" (M. Panjabi). *European Spine Journal, 16*(10), 1733–1735.

Schoenheimer, R. (1942). *The Dynamic State of Body Constituents.* Cambridge, MA: Harvard University Press.

Selye, H. (1976). *The Stress of Life.* New York, NY: McGraw-Hill.

Sheets-Johnstone, M. (Ed.). (1992). *Giving the Body Its Due.* Albany, NY: SUNY Press.

Siegel, D. (1999). *The Developing Mind: Toward a Neurobiology of Interpersonal Experience.* New York, NY: Guilford Press.

Siegel, D. (2010). *Mindsight: The New Science of Personal Transformation.* New York, NY: Bantam Books.

Solomon, G. (1993). An Important Theoretical Advance. *Advances, 9*(2), 31–39.

Squotas-Emch, S. A., Glaser, R., & Kiecolt-Glaser, J. (1992). No. 155–178. Psychological Influences on Immune and Endocrine Function. In F. H. Willard & M. Patterson (Eds.), *Nociception and the Neuroindocrine-Immune Connection* (pp. 294–312). Athens, OH: University Classics.

Stecco, C., Gagey, O., Belloni, A., Pozzuoli, A., Porzionato, A., Macchi, V., et al. (2007). Anatomy of the Deep Fascia of the Upper Limb. Second Part: Study of Innervation. *Morphologie, 91*(292), 38–43.

Taylor, K. (1995). *The Ethics of Caring, Honoring the Web of Life in Our Professional Healing Relationships* (2nd ed.). Santa Cruz, CA: Hanford Mead Publishers.

Trager, M., Guadagno-Hammond, C., & Turnley Walker, T. (1987). *Trager Mentastics: Movement as a Way to Agelessness.* Barrytown, NY: Station Hill Press.

Travell, J. G., & Simons, D. G. (1992). *Myofascial Pain and Dysfunction: The Trigger Point Manual: Vol. 2 The Lower Extremities.* Philadelphia, PA: Lippincott Williams & Wilkins.

Travell, J. G., & Simons, D. G. (1998). *Myofascial Pain and Dysfunction: The Trigger Point Manual: Vol. 1 The Upper Half of the Body* (2nd ed.). Los Angeles, CA: Lippincott Williams & Wilkins.

Trungpa, C. (1980). Becoming a Full Human Being. *Naropa Institute Journal of Psychology, 1*, 4–20.

Van der Kolk, B. (Producer). (2012). *How Trauma Traps Survivors in the Past—A Look at Trauma Therapy.*

Varela, F., Thompson, E., & Rosch, E. (1992). *The Embodied Mind: Cognitive Science and Human Experience.* Cambridge, MA: MIT Press.

Ward, R. C. (1993). Myofascial Release Concepts. In J. V. Basmajian & R. E. Nyberg (Eds.), *Rational Manual Therapies.* Baltimore, MD: Lippincott Williams & Wilkins.

Weiner, H. (1992). *Perturbing the Organism.* Chicago, IL: University of Chicago Press.

Willard, F. H., & Patterson, M. M. (1992). *Nociception and the Neuroendocrine-Immune Connection.* Paper presented at the 1992 International Symposium.

Wolfstein, B. (Ed.). (1998). *Essential Papers on Counter-Transference.* New York, NY: New York University Press.

INDEX

N

O

P

Q

R

T

U

V

ACKNOWLEDGEMENTS

Holly Pinto

If you are lucky, the perfect teacher will come into your life and make an incredible difference in your life. I got lucky. Dr. Michael Shea has been my teacher, my mentor, and my friend for the past 25 years. From my whole heart, I thank you. I thank you for everything you have taught me. You have influenced and enriched my life in so many ways. You have been an inspiration to me, and I am the massage therapist and school owner that I am today because of you. I am grateful to have you in my life.

I have used your original manuals as a student, as a therapist, and as a school owner over a span of 25 years. They are timeless, and the information in them is as good today as it was back then. Thank you for including me in the effort of rebirthing these manuals.

Thank you to Angela Banks, my assistant and an incredible therapist, for the endless hours of editing and proofing. I could not have done this without your help, patience, love, and support. You are amazing.

To my students Rodney, Patti, Jessica, Mindy, Alicia, Amanda, La-Nell, Brandy, Martha, Jen, and Mikaela, thank you for all of your wonderful feedback.

To Wendy, my photographer, and Martha, my model, thank you.

To my sisters, Candi Hamill and Vicki Cameron, thank you for being my cheerleaders. I get my strength and courage from you both.

I am inspired every day to do better because of my two beautiful girls, Amy Lorraine and Stephanie Lauren. You two are the true loves of my life.

To my loyal staff, Tammy Bivin, Nick Gephart, and Angela Banks, I could not do it without you. A special thanks to Dr. Gary Rovin and Dr. Daniel Rovin for all of the support and love that you have given me throughout the years. You are the best. Your knowledge of the body is exceptional and I have learned so much from all of you. Dr. Ashley Gaines, a very special thank you to you as well.

To Don Kelley, CNMT, my NMT instructor. Thank you for sharing all of your incredible knowledge with me and my staff. Not to mention your humor! We are very grateful to you and Judith DeLany.

I am so grateful that I get to get up and do what I do every day. My passion and love for this work has remained strong. I adore my little schoolhouse and everything it stands for. It is my students who make it what it is. You are everything. You teach me something new every day. This manual is for you.

Michael Shea

First I would like to acknowledge my wife Cathy and her great generosity in being the model for most of the photographs in this volume. Cathy and I met in 1987, and I began having these therapeutic skills photographed even before we were married. The photographer Claudine Laabs is one of the premier nature photographers in South Florida. Almost all of the photographs were taken outside in natural lighting. As the viewer can see, the photographs were taken over a period of several years as I developed my teaching. There is a very pleasing aesthetic that Claudine provides with her work.

I am grateful to all my teachers at the Rolf Institute because I know now that I was a tough nut to crack. One teacher in particular stood out, and his name was Peter Melchior. Peter eventually asked me to be an assistant in his training, and I spent a lot of time receiving work from him, getting to know him, and learning to love him as one of the most gifted Rolfers in the world. I am also grateful to my first Rolfer, Jim Asher. As a requirement to enter the Rolf Institute, I had to receive the Rolfing series and then get a recommendation from that person. Jim mentored me in so many ways as I started my career back in 1979. My brother Brian also went through the Rolf Institute training, and I must say that there is nothing better in the whole wide world than to share body work with a brother. I had many other brothers in the Rolf Institute, such as Bill Smythe and Ray McCall. I had sisters as well, Heather Wing and Megan James. All of these people helped me in so many ways with such great kindness and humor. Finally I want to acknowledge my friend Valerie Caruso who is an expert in myofascial release and edited the early versions of this book.

ABOUT THE AUTHORS

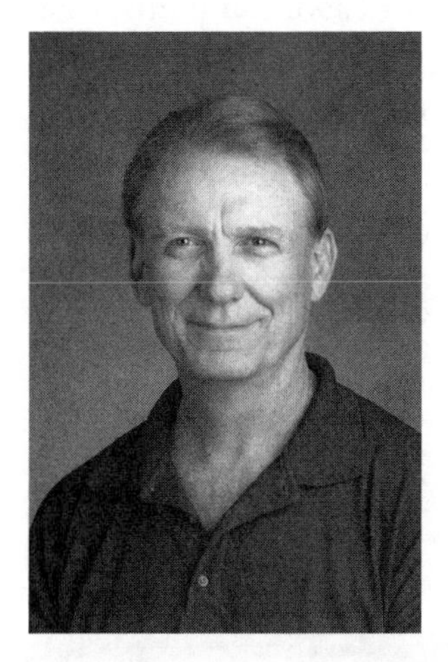

One of the Upledger Institute's first certified full instructors of craniosacral therapy in 1986, Michael Shea, Ph.D., has taught somatic psychology, myofascial release, visceral manipulation, and biodynamic craniosacral therapy worldwide for more than 35 years. He is cofounder of the International Affiliation of Biodynamic Trainings, a founding board member of the Biodynamic Craniosacral Therapy Association of North America, and a student of His Holiness the Dalai Lama. Dr. Shea has also taught human embryology and fetal-placental development in the somatic psychology and pre- and perinatal doctoral programs at the Santa Barbara Graduate Institute and has served on several pre- and perinatal psychology doctoral committees. He lives in Juno Beach, Florida, with his wife, Cathy. For more information on his courses and trainings, visit www.michaelsheateaching.com.

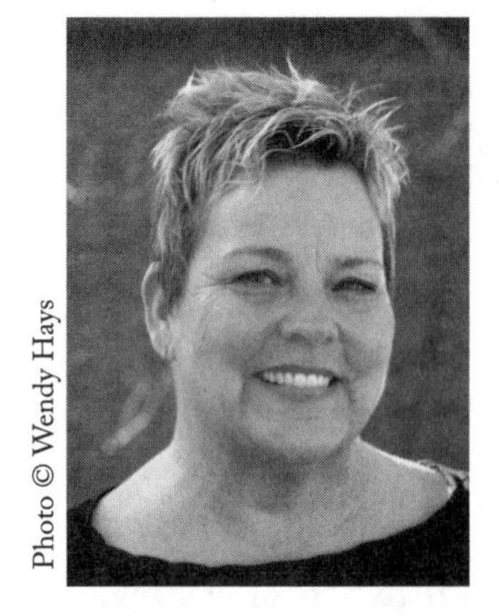
Photo © Wendy Hays

Holly Pinto, BS, LMT, BCTMB, is the founder and director of the Body Therapy Center and School of Massage which has operated in Swansea, Illinois since 1997. Holly is a graduate of the Neuromuscular Concepts School of Massage in San Antonio, Texas. Her specialties in addition to massage include myofascial release, neuromuscular therapy, WATSU/waterdance, and biodynamic craniosacral therapy. Holly is an instructor for Judith DeLany's neuromuscular therapy American version in her school program. She has been a member of the American Massage Therapy Association since 1991 and was certified by the National Certification Board of Therapeutic Massage and Bodywork in 1994. Holly continues to teach and work a private practice.